Managing Health Services

Understanding Public Health

Series editors: Nick Black and Rosalind Raine, London School of Hygiene & Tropical Medicine

Throughout the world, recognition of the importance of public health to sustainable, safe and healthy societies is growing. The achievements of public health in nineteenth-century Europe were for much of the twentieth century overshadowed by advances in personal care, in particular in hospital care. Now, with the dawning of a new century, there is increasing understanding of the inevitable limits of individual health care and of the need to complement such services with effective public health strategies. Major improvements in people's health will come from controlling communicable diseases, eradicating environmental hazards, improving people's diets and enhancing the availability and quality of effective health care. To achieve this, every country needs a cadre of knowledgeable public health practitioners with social, political and organizational skills to lead and bring about changes at international, national and local levels.

This is one of a series of 20 books that provides a foundation for those wishing to join in and contribute to the twenty-first-century regeneration of public health, helping to put the concerns and perspectives of public health at the heart of policy-making and service provision. While each book stands alone, together they provide a comprehensive account of the three main aims of public health: protecting the public from environmental hazards, improving the health of the public and ensuring high quality health services are available to all. Some of the books focus on methods, others on key topics. They have been written by staff at the London School of Hygiene & Tropical Medicine with considerable experience of teaching public health to students from low-, middle- and high-income countries. Much of the material has been developed and tested with postgraduate students both in face-to-face teaching and through distance learning.

The books are designed for self-directed learning. Each chapter has explicit learning objectives, key terms are highlighted and the text contains many activities to enable the reader to test their own understanding of the ideas and material covered. Written in a clear and accessible style, the series will be essential reading for students taking postgraduate courses in public health and will also be of interest to public health practitioners and policy-makers.

Titles in the series

Analytical models for decision making: Colin Sanderson and Reinhold Gruen
Controlling communicable disease: Norman Noah
Economic analysis for management and policy: Stephen Jan, Lilani Kumaranayake, Jenny Roberts, Kara Hanson and Kate Archibald
Economic evaluation: Julia Fox-Rushby and John Cairns (eds)
Environmental epidemiology: Paul Wilkinson (ed.)
Environment, health and sustainable development: Megan Landon
Environmental health policy: David Ball (ed.)
Financial management in health services: Reinhold Gruen and Anne Howarth
Global change and health: Kelley Lee and Jeff Collin (eds)
Health care evaluation: Sarah Smith, Don Sinclair, Rosalind Raine and Barnaby Reeves
Health promotion practice: Maggie Davies, Wendy Macdowall and Chris Bonell (eds)
Health promotion theory: Maggie Davies and Wendy Macdowall (eds)
Introduction to epidemiology: Lucianne Bailey, Katerina Vardulaki, Julia Langham and Daniel Chandramohan
Introduction to health economics: David Wonderling, Reinhold Gruen and Nick Black
Issues in public health: Joceline Pomerleau and Martin McKee (eds)
Making health policy: Kent Buse, Nicholas Mays and Gill Walt
Managing health services: Nick Goodwin, Reinhold Gruen and Valerie Iles
Medical anthropology: Robert Pool and Wenzel Geissler
Principles of social research: Judith Green and John Browne (eds)
Understanding health services: Nick Black and Reinhold Gruen

Managing Health Services

Nick Goodwin, Reinhold Gruen
and Valerie Iles

Open University Press

Open University Press
McGraw-Hill Education
McGraw-Hill House
Shoppenhangers Road
Maidenhead
Berkshire
England
SL6 2QL

email: enquiries@openup.co.uk
world wide web: www.openup.co.uk

and Two Penn Plaza, New York, NY 10121-2289, USA

First published 2006

A catalogue record of this book is available from the British Library

ISBN-10: 0 335 218510
ISBN-13: 978 0 335 218523

Library of Congress Cataloging-in-Publication Data
CIP data has been applied for

Typeset by RefineCatch Limited, Bungay, Suffolk
Printed in the UK by Bell & Bain Ltd, Glasgow

Contents

Acknowledgements

Open University Press and the London School of Hygiene & Tropical Medicine have made every effort to obtain permission from copyright holders to reproduce material in this book and to acknowledge these sources correctly. Any omissions brought to our attention will be remedied in future editions.

We would like to express our grateful thanks to the following copyright holders for granting permission to reproduce material in this book.

p. 175   Ackerman L, 'Development, transition or transformation: the question of change in organizations,' in J Hoy, D van Eynde and DC van Eynde, *Organization Development Classics*, 1997, Copyright John Wiley and Sons.

p. 215   Blake Robert, and Mouton Jane, *The New Managerial Grid III: The Key to Leadership Excellence*, 1985, Gulf Publishing Company. Copyright Grid International Inc.

p. 55, 57   Bobadilla JL, Cowley P, Musgrove P and Saxenian, 'Design, content and financing of an essential national package of health services,' *Bulletin of the World Health Organization*, 1994, 72: 653–662. Reprinted with permission from World Health Organization.

p. 88   This material is taken from 'Practical Manpower Planning' by M Brahman, 1988, with the permission of the publisher, the Chartered Institute of Personnel and Development, London.

p. 189   Checkland P and Scholes J, *Soft Systems Methodology in Action*, 1999. Copyright John Wiley and Sons Ltd. Reproduced with permission.

p. 129, 151 W. Edwards Deming, *Out of Crisis*, published by The MIT Press. Copyright © 1986, The MIT Press.

p. 216, 218 Fiedler FE, *A Theory of Leadership Effectiveness*, McGraw-Hill Publishing. © 1967 Fred E Fiedler, reprinted by permission of Fred E Fiedler.

p. 178   Fombrun C, Tichy N and Devanna M, *Strategic Human Resource Management*. Copyright © 1984, John Wiley and Sons. Reprinted with permission of John Wiley & Sons, Inc.

p. 109   Freeman RE, 'Strategic management: a stakeholder approach,' 1984, Financial Times Prentice Hall. © R Edward Freeman 1984, reprinted with permission from R Edward Freeman.

p. 73   Guest D, 'Personnel and HRM: Can you tell the difference?,' *People Management*, January 1989, 21(1): 48–51. Reproduced with permission.

p. 114   *The Herald*, Zimbabwe, 1985.

p. 220–1   Hersey P (1984) 'The Situational Leader', p63. Reprinted with permission of the Center for Leadership Studies, Inc. Escondido, CA, USA. All rights reserved.

p. 175   Provided by Kate Grimes in Iles V and Sutherland K, 'Managing Change in the NHS,' 2001. NCCSDO.

p. 149   Portions of these materials are copyrighted by Oriel Incorporated, formerly Joiner Associates Inc and are used here with permission. Further reproductions are prohibited without written consent of Oriel Incorporated. Call 1–800–669–8326.

p. 24   Katz R, 'Skills of an effective administrator,' Harvard Business Review, 1955, 33: 33–42. Reprinted with permission.

p. 32   La Monica E and Morgan P, 'Management in health care: a theoretical and experiential approach,' 1994 Palgrave Macmillan, reproduced with permission of Palgrave Macmillan.

p. 192   Based on Lewin, K. 1997, *Resolving Social Conflicts and Field Theory in Social Science*. Washington D.C: American Psychological Association.

p. 18   Mintzberg H, *Mintzberg on Management* (1989), Hungry Minds Inc, US.

p. 39, 40   Mossialos E, Dixon A, Figueras J, Kutzin J (eds), *Funding Health Care:*
41, 42   *Options for Europe*. © 2002, Open University Press. Reproduced with the kind permission of the Open University Press.

p. 16   Mullins LJ, *Management and Organizational Behaviour*, 5th edition, Pearson Education Limited. © Laurie J Mullins, 1985, 1989, 1993, 1996, 1999.

p. 26   Pedler M, Burgoyne J and Boydell T, *A Manager's Guide to Self Development*, 3rd edn. © 1994, McGraw-Hill Publishing Company. Reproduced with the kind permission of McGraw-Hill Publishing Company.

p. 186   McKinsey 7-S Framework (diagram, p10) from *In Search of Excellence: Lessons from America's Best Run Companies* by Thomas J. Peters and Robert H. Waterman, Jr. Copyright © 1982 Thomas J. Peters and Robert H. Waterman, Jr. Reprinted by permission of HarperCollins Publishers.

p. 89   Strike Anthony J, *Human Resources in Health Care: A Manager's Guide*, Blackwell Publishing Ltd, 1995. Reprinted with permission.

p. 77   Warner M, 'Human Resource Management "with Chinese characteristics"', *The International Journal of Human Resource Management*, 1995, 4(1) with permission from Taylor and Francis Ltd. http://www.tandf.co.uk/journals.

p. 47, 49,   World Health Organization, *The World Health Report 2000. Health*
51, 60, 62,   *systems: improving performance, 2000*.
63, 64

p. 208   Yukl GA, *Leadership in Organizations*, 2nd Edition, © 1989. Adapted by permission of Pearson Education, Inc., Upper Saddle River, NJ.

Overview of the book

Introduction

Health care systems around the world are highly complex and dynamic. Their characteristics differ greatly across a range of dimensions, including the level of state regulation; the methods for health care commissioning and delivery; the level of competition between health care providers; and the financial mechanisms through which health systems are funded. Different health care systems influence the way these tasks are managed, yet, regardless of these differences, the need for effective managers and managerial leaders is essential in allowing organizations and professionals to achieve specific goals.

This book covers the key issues involved in health services management. It examines and unpicks the concepts of management, health care funding, human resource management, performance management, change management and managerial leadership in the context of delivering effective health care services. It provides an understanding, both theoretical and practical, of the managerial processes and skills that are required to achieve these tasks.

Why study health services management?

It is widely recognized that effective management and leadership are essential if health care professionals and managers are to fulfil their responsibilities, both to themselves and also to the users of health services. It is important, therefore, that the role of managers in health services is understood and that management theories and techniques are recognized so they may be adopted in practice.

Structure of the book

The book contains nineteen chapters in six sections, as shown on the contents page. Each chapter includes:

- an overview,
- a list of learning objectives,
- a list of key terms,
- a range of activities,
- feedback on activities,
- a summary.

The examples provided in the book are balanced between high-, middle- and low-income countries. However, you should be aware that much of the theory on health services management is drawn from high-income countries. The following description of the section and chapter contents will give you an idea of what you will be studying.

Understanding the roles of managers and management in health care

The first section of this book introduces the concept of management and how to apply the generic tasks of management effectively in the context of health service delivery. In Chapter 1, you will consider the basics of good management and understand three fundamental 'rules' of managing in health care that will form the basis of your approach to management. Chapter 2 sets out the general process of management, including an examination of roles and role theory. The chapter contrasts key differences in the role of health service managers in the public sector with those in industry and the private sector, as well as between high- and low-income countries. In Chapter 3, a picture of the core qualities required of the manager in health services is developed, including an appreciation of how managerial roles in health care are changing. Chapter 4 examines how accomplishing goals requires a conscious, identifiable strategy – a framework known as the 'problem-solving method'. Case study activities will show you how to adopt such methods in practice.

Health care funding

Management text books often tend to miss out the implications for managers of the way services are financed and purchased. In this section you will address this by reviewing the key functions involved in funding and purchasing health services and the implications for managers. Chapter 5 provides an international analysis of how revenue is collected (general taxation, social insurance, private insurance and direct payments), how funds are pooled, and how care is then purchased from providers. Chapter 6 then examines the three fundamental management challenges to purchasing health services: deciding what to purchase, from whom, and how.

Managing people

The third section explores a key aspect of health services management – the management and development of staff in health care organizations. It will enable you to adapt the techniques learned here to your own health care organizations. Chapter 7 begins by presenting the principal activities and tools of human resource management with particular emphasis on the strategic human resource management cycle and its application both in the public and the private sectors. Chapter 8 examines human resource planning, including the forecasting of demand. Chapter 9 tackles recruitment and selection, including the influence of corruption, nepotism and discrimination in personnel procedures. Chapter 10 considers methods of performance management, appraisal and training, while Chapter 11 introduces the issues and potential problems involved in managing interprofessional groups.

Managing results

This section examines how managers develop indicators and collect information to determine the extent to which health care organizations are meeting their objectives. It aims to provide an overview of the purpose of performance management in organizations and discusses the problem of developing output indicators in the public sector where performance indicators almost universally exclude a consideration of profit. Using a systems approach, the section summarizes levels of results and how to interpret and manage these results.

Chapter 12 presents the purpose and principles of performance management in organizations and examines the different ways performance can be measured in terms of the efficiency of processes. Chapter 13 takes the debate forward by examining how quality can be measured and managed to improve health services delivery. Chapter 14 examines the use of pay structures in improving organizational performance, specifically the use of performance-related pay.

Managing change

This section examines how managers can assess the need for change as well as manage the process of change. In Chapter 15, you will first consider the importance of creating a sense of organizational purpose in planning and achieving goals before assessing the role of strategic management. Chapter 16 provides an introduction to change management in health services and discusses its key terms and concepts. Building on previous chapters, it summarizes the role of human resources management in offering an integrated approach to managing and developing people in the context of a changing public sector environment. An empirical model is developed that enables you to apply design criteria for managing change. In particular, the chapter focuses on organizational culture and how this can be managed. Chapter 17 presents and assesses some of the main tools and models that managers can use to make change happen.

The leadership role of managers

Whatever the organizational context, the role of a manager is ultimately about leadership. In Chapter 18, approaches to leadership and the nature of power are examined, in order to gain an understanding of the key qualities of a leader. Chapter 19 shows how the different styles of leadership adopted can have a significant impact on the motivation of staff in meeting organizational goals.

Acknowledgements

The authors would like to acknowledge the important contributions made by Willy McCourt and Derek Eldridge (Chapters 7–10, 12, 14, 16) who developed teaching material for the London School of Hygiene & Tropical Medicine on which some of the content of this book is founded. We thank Deirdre Byrne, series manager, for her help and support.

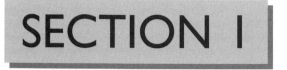

SECTION I

Understanding the roles of managers and management in health care

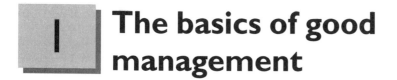

The basics of good management

Overview

There are many core activities that a manager must undertake. In this introductory chapter, you will consider the basics of good management and understand three ways of improving your performance as a manager – the so-called 'fundamental rules' of management. They should form the basis of your approach to management.

Learning objectives

After working through this chapter you will be able to:

- **describe three fundamental 'rules' for managing others;**
- **discuss means of implementing these rules;**
- **consider how to apply the rules in your own service.**

Key terms

Complicated easy management concepts Concepts that are mastered using intelligence and, once mastered, require only intelligence to implement.

Simple hard management concepts Concepts that are simple to understand but require courage and discipline to implement.

The three fundamental 'rules' of management

Valerie Iles (1997) has suggested three fundamental 'rules' for managing people in health care:

Rule 1: Agree with them precisely what it is you expect them to achieve.
Rule 2: Ensure both you and they are confident that they have the skills and resources to achieve it.
Rule 3: Give them feedback on whether they are achieving it.

The first 'rule' reflects that people will go about different tasks in different ways – some may be so fastidious that they miss deadlines; others may go off in a different direction to the task at hand. Some people may be responsive to being 'told' what to do, others need to feel engaged in the decision-making process itself. Agreeing, managing and renewing expectations is thus a key managerial task requiring both parties to express their views, probably at a face-to-face level.

Iles' second 'rule' is concerned with ensuring that both managers and those being managed are confident they can achieve the task and have the necessary skills, expertise and resources available. The process cannot necessarily be pre-determined, since the skills for some tasks only become apparent as the nature of the work is revealed. However, matching skills and expectations is important in the ability of an individual or team to perform their tasks.

The third 'rule' concerns the process of giving feedback to ensure that people know that goals are being reached or not and whether extra effort or a different approach is required. Feedback is fundamental because it is only by receiving feedback from others that skills can be improved and developed. You probably understand this and may feel this is obvious, but Iles argues that it is as much the attitude, as the frequency, of feedback that matters.

The following scenario illustrates these rules.

The Johnson family

The Johnson family recently decided to employ a cleaner in their home. They were pleased when Mrs White replied to their advertisement. She had good references from other clients and seemed friendly and likeable. They asked her to start the next day. With both Mr and Mrs Johnson out at work, Mrs White worked on her own without any supervision. At first the Johnsons were delighted to come home to a tidy house, but after a few weeks Mrs Johnson noticed that the kitchen cupboards were rather dirty, that the floor hadn't been swept in the corners and that the fridge needed defrosting. She arranged to leave work early to speak to Mrs White and told her that she wanted her to be much more thorough in her cleaning.

A few weeks later things were no better and the Johnsons were upset to find that Mrs White had broken one of their valuable porcelain ornaments. 'Why did you touch it?' they asked her. 'We keep all our porcelain figures in that cabinet especially so that they don't need cleaning.' They also told her, rather angrily, that they were still unhappy with her work. Mrs White told them to find another cleaner.

At a friend's house, soon afterwards, Mrs Johnson was introduced to one of the people who had written a reference for Mrs White. In conversation she was amazed to hear how thorough and careful Mrs White had been with this other client. 'But she was so careless for us', she exclaimed. 'She never once defrosted the fridge, nor cleaned inside the kitchen cupboards.' 'I don't suppose she did; I would never dream of asking a cleaner to do that', the other woman replied.

Discussing this incident with her friend later, Mrs Johnson wondered aloud how she had ever assumed Mrs White would know what they wanted of her. 'I think I felt it would be an insult to her; it would be questioning her competence, a demonstration that we didn't trust her', she said. Her friend asked why she had not told her once it was clear there was a problem. Mrs Johnson replied, 'I suppose I didn't want to hurt her feelings . . . I wanted to be nice.'

Activity 1.1

1 Rule number one: *agree with them precisely what it is you expect them to achieve.*

   (a) Did the Johnsons implement rule number one?
   (b) What should they have said to Mrs White to make sure that she knew what they wanted her to do?

2 Rule number two: *ensure that both you and they are confident that they have the skills and resources to achieve it.*

   (a) Did the Johnsons implement rule number two?
   (b) What should they have done to ensure that their fragile and valuable ornaments would be expertly looked after?

3 Rule number three: *give them feedback on whether they are achieving it.*

   (a) Did the Johnsons implement rule number three?
   (b) What was wrong with the feedback Mrs Johnson gave to Mrs White?

4 If the Johnsons had explained exactly how they wanted their house cleaned, would this have demonstrated that they did not trust Mrs White? Why?

5 Mrs Johnson says that she didn't want to hurt Mrs White's feelings and that she wanted to be nice. Whose feelings is she most concerned about? What does she mean by 'I wanted to be nice'?

Feedback

The Johnsons did not implement any of the three 'rules'.

1 They did not tell Mrs White how they wanted her to clean the floor, that they expected her to clean inside the cupboards, nor that she should defrost the fridge. Everyone has different ways of doing things and so they must make their wishes known. Mrs Johnson was not wrong to want Mrs White to do these things; but she was wrong to expect her to know them without being told.

2 The Johnsons did not check that Mrs White would recognize valuable porcelain and treat it differently from other items in the house.

3 Mrs Johnson told Mrs White to 'be more thorough'. Imagine you are Mrs White and you are trying hard to please Mrs Johnson. When she tells you to 'be more thorough', what do you do? You probably work harder at the things you are already doing. You certainly do not decide to defrost the fridge if you have no idea you are expected to do so. In other words, Mrs Johnson was not specific enough in her feedback for it to be useful.

4 The Johnsons want their home cleaned in a particular way. It does not demonstrate a lack of trust in a cleaner if they explain what they want. In any case, trust has to be earned.

5 Mrs Johnson is more concerned about her own feelings than she is about those of Mrs White. By 'being nice' she probably means: 'I wanted her to like me and think I'm a nice person'.

Aim for respect rather than popularity

Often when people say, or think, that they do not want to hurt someone else's feelings, it is their own feelings they are most concerned about: feelings of embarrassment, of discomfort, a fear of not being liked, of not knowing what to say if the other person becomes angry or upset, a desire not to get into an argument. It is for this reason that many people prefer to write a complaint rather than deal with it face to face. If you have a genuine concern for the other person, then you will want to give them the information they need in order to be successful in their role. They may not always appreciate it, particularly at the time, but you will have given them the opportunity to improve and do better for themselves.

Being 'nice' is often associated with self-interest, with wanting to be liked, and not with concern for the other person or for the service. Managers, then, should not try to be nice but to be fair, flexible, open-minded and courageous. They should aim to be respected rather than liked. And, indeed, trying to be liked is a self-defeating aim; most managers who try to be nice are neither liked nor respected.

Implementing these rules for yourself

If you implement these rules yourself, you will have staff who know what you expect them to do, you will be confident that they can do it and you will become more and more skilful at influencing their performance by giving them feedback. Although, so far, you have considered these three rules only in the context of a manager and a subordinate, they can often be useful in relationships between colleagues.

✐ Activity 1.2

Think of a staff team you have managed. If you do not have a team of people whom you manage then think instead of colleagues or people you may manage in a voluntary capacity in your community.

On a sheet of paper turned sideways (landscape) write down the following headings at the top:

- Team member
- Expectations
- Agreed with them?
- Skills and resources required by team member
- Skills and resources they have
- Date of last feedback

Think of your own immediate staff team. Write their names in the first column, spacing them out so that you allow for three or four lines of writing for each.

Do you think you are applying all of the three rules with each of these people? Yes/No

For each of the people you have listed, write down in the second column what you expect them to achieve. In the third column, put a tick by the achievements you think they know about and agree with.

Now in column four, list the skills and resources that they need if they are to meet your expectations, and in the fifth column tick those which they have. In this column you can also put a cross alongside the skills they do not have and a query where you are uncertain whether they have the necessary skills and resources.

Against each name write down the date when you last gave them feedback on their performance. Do this for the last time you gave them feedback on each of your expectations. Complete this chart for at least three people.

↻ Feedback

Your entries in your completed chart will be unique to the roles and responsibilities within your team. The example in Table 1.1 shows how the chart might have been completed for Sally Brown, a member of a community nursing team.

Table 1.1 Examples of assessment of team members

Team member	Expectations	Agreed with them?	Skills and resources required by team member	Skills and resources they have	Date of last feedback
Sally Brown	1 visit at least five patients in their homes every working day	✓	1a professional skills of assessment and treatment	✓	20/08
			1b access to transport	✓	
			1c scheduling skills	✗	
			1d recording system	✓	
	2 attend weekly team meeting	✓	2a dates and times of meetings	✗	15/06
	3 support other members of the community team	✓	3a information about skills of other team members	✗	never
			3b information about caseloads of other team members	✗	
			3c forum for discussing support needed	✗	
	4 provide information on activities to managers		4a information system	✓	last year
			4b skills in using any technology needed	✓	
			4c time to enter data	?	
	5 arrive promptly at 9.00am	✓	5a punctuality	✓	23/08
	6 keep up to date clinically		6a clinical audit system	✓	20/08
			6b access to journals	✓	
			6c skills in reflection and evaluation of own practice	?	

Most managers would not be able to put ticks in all the boxes, indeed many would only be able to enter a few, if they were honest. So do not feel disheartened if you, too, are unable to do so. However, turning your attention to how you can implement the three rules with these people you will have to engage with your staff face to face. This will require you to be both clear-thinking and, perhaps, courageous. It is not always easy to start a discussion about your expectations with someone who has been in post for a long time and whose behaviour or performance no one has challenged before. So develop an *action plan* and have some personal support mechanisms – perhaps a friend or colleague you can discuss it with.

Activity 1.3

You have read at the beginning of this chapter the guidelines for giving and receiving feedback. Now try putting them into practice. Call to mind one member of your team to whom you feel you should give some feedback. It could be about something they are doing, something they have done, or something they are not doing. Use the guidelines to prepare what you will say, where and how. Ask a friend to comment on how well you are observing the guidelines.

Feedback

Giving feedback to colleagues needs to be constructive and involve a two-way dialogue in which views can be shared and agreements reached. In your preparations, you should have attempted to follow the three rules: first, agreeing (or reviewing) expectations for the task; second, discussing whether the necessary resources or skills are in place to achieve the task; and third, giving feedback on their performance. At the end of the discussion a clearly agreed set of actions should have been decided upon and understood.

The 'simple hard' and the 'complicated easy'

Many people believe that to become a good manager you need to learn new skills. That is true, but there is more to it than that. You also need to develop new ways of behaving. This chapter has been all about the 'simple hard'. It has introduced three rules which are simple to state, easy to remember, but hard to observe. People who have been brought up to value the 'complicated easy', and that includes many health care professionals, often dislike the simple hard. They do so for two reasons.

First, it is simple. The complicated easy is more intellectually satisfying, and there is a tendency to dismiss what is simple as 'simplistic'. Second, it is hard. Once you have grasped the concepts of the complicated easy, you can apply them immediately. Your ease of doing so will increase with experience, but it is possible to use them well as soon as you have properly understood them. Not so the simple hard. Implementing these takes much practice, much experience and reflection on that experience. Implementing the simple hard is as much to do with integrity as it is with intellect.

Of course, *both* the simple hard and the complicated easy are essential for health care managers. Both are necessary, neither alone is sufficient. It is also the case that, such are the pressures on health care organizations that the complicated easy aspects are indeed very complicated, and do not feel at all easy. The distinction is that, although they require very considerable intellectual capacity, that is all they require. The simple hard call on our behaviours, our feelings, our integrity.

Summary

There are three tasks of such fundamental importance to managing other people effectively that you can think of them as rules. The rules are: agree with them precisely what it is you expect them to achieve; ensure that both you and they are confident that they have the skills and resources to achieve it; and give them feedback on whether they are achieving it.

Understanding the three rules is simple, but they are hard to put into practice because they require time, energy and courage. Good management requires an understanding of two types of concepts: those that are complicated but easy to implement because they involve brains but not emotions, and simple hard concepts, like the three rules, which require more courage and discipline than intelligence.

Reference

Iles, V. (1997) *Really Managing Health Care*. Buckingham: Open University Press.

2 The nature of management

Overview

In this chapter you will learn about the nature of managerial work and how to set out the general process of management, including roles and role theory. The chapter contrasts key differences in the role of health service managers in the public sector with those in the private sector, as well as between high- and low-income countries.

Learning objectives

After working through this chapter you will be able to:

- explain the meaning of management and understand its main roles and functions;
- recognize the key components of role theory;
- understand why organizations need managers;
- describe key differences between management tasks in health services in the public sector and those in the private sector;
- describe key differences in the managerial tasks faced by managers in low-income countries compared to high-income countries.

Key terms

Classical management theory A scientifically based approach to the practice of management involving tasks and functions.

Decisional roles Managerial roles at the 'front line', including dealing with disputes, negotiating with staff, allocating resources and initiating change.

Informational roles Managerial roles based on fulfilling interpersonal goals, including monitoring activity, disseminating information and dealing with the concerns of key stakeholders.

Interpersonal roles Managerial roles based on formal authority, including leadership, liaison with external organizations and acting as a figurehead.

New public management An approach to government involving the application of private sector management techniques.

Role theory A role-based analysis of managerial tasks, originating with the work of Mintzberg, which examines observed roles as opposed to prescribed tasks.

The nature of management – as much art as science

Health services can only achieve their goals through the coordinated efforts of a wide range of staff. It is the task of management to get this work done by influencing the actions of other people through the integration of activities. As you work through this book, you will begin to appreciate that management is not just, as so-called classical theorists such as Taylor (1911) and Fayol (1949) suggested, a scientifically based discipline that can be based on standardized rules and formulae. Rather, management is also about understanding personal behaviours in order to 'get things done through other people' (Dale, 1965). Peter Drucker, a leading management guru, argued that the ultimate test of management is the achievement of optimum organizational performance measured by achievable objectives (Drucker, 1977).

What do managers do?

Many authors have discussed the process components, or common activities, of management. One of the most widely quoted is Henri Fayol (1949), who analysed the activities in industry to arrive at six key groups:

- *Technical* – production, manufacture and adaptation
- *Commercial* – buying, selling and exchanging market information
- *Financial* – obtaining capital and making optimum use of funds
- *Security* – safeguarding property and person
- *Accounting* – stocktaking and balancing costs
- *Managerial* – which Fayol further describes has five elements:
  1 *Planning* – examining future needs and developing a plan of action
  2 *Organizing* – providing human resources and capital to carry out organizational activities
  3 *Command* – getting the optimum from employees to the goals of the organization
  4 *Co-ordination* – unifying and harmonizing activities to facilitate successful working
  5 *Control* – verifying that plans are being adhered to through commands

Many other writers have since analysed the elements of management and each shows a basic similarity. Brech's (1975) principles of management, for example, emphasize management as a 'social process' and adds 'motivation', or the ability to inspire morale, onto the list of managerial tasks created by Fayol. Drucker (1977) identifies further the needs of a manager to develop and train people as well as to establish performance criteria on which to judge individual and group performance.

A synthesis of the roles of managers by Mullins (1999) distinguishes between those managers whose key occupation is to 'perform tasks' with those that determine how and where these tasks should be performed. His summary of the essential nature of managerial work (Figure 2.1) is a helpful visual interpretation of these differences, which emphasizes the wide range of management practices and management styles that exist.

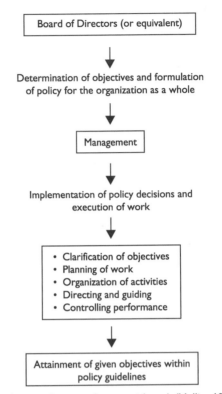

Figure 2.1 Summary of essential nature of managerial work (Mullins 1999)

Mintzberg's role theory

Mintzberg (1989), another of the gurus of management, argued that much of the above analysis of management tasks and skills does not really help us to understand what managers really do. None of the writings, he argued, distinguished between 'ideals' (what a manager *should* do) and 'images' (what a manager is *observed* doing). For example, in an international study of foremen, factory supervisors, staff managers, sales managers, hospital administrators, company presidents and even street-gang leaders – across the United States, Canada, Sweden and Great Britain – Mintzberg paints a very different picture to that of the rational or 'scientific' manager. He uncovered four 'myths' about management and concluded that a manager's role can more accurately be described as a set of ten 'roles' or 'behaviours'.

Activity 2.1

Thinking about your role as a manager, or those of the managers where you work, attempt to make a distinction between what you think the manager is supposed to be doing (in terms of the key activities described above), and the roles that the manager actually does.

1   Can you guess the four managerial 'myths' that were uncovered by Mintzberg?
2   Develop a list of 'real' roles that a manager plays on a daily basis – to what extent are these based on the application of formal authority, the giving of information, or the undertaking of interpersonal relationships?

Feedback

1   You may have found legitimate alternative answers, but you might have identified one or more of the following myths:

*   Managers are often not rational planners who think ahead; their decision-making is often characterized by intuition, discontinuity and a dislike of reflection.
*   Managers spend little time actually managing operational activities but more time negotiating with staff, developing and providing information, and holding meetings.
*   Managers tend not to rely on aggregated or quantified data on which to make decisions, but tend to rely more on information such as gossip, hearsay and speculation. Much information of high value is never written down, so informal channels of communication may be the most important source of data.
*   Management is not solely a scientific task, but involves a considerable amount of judgement and intuition.

2   As a result of his analyses, Mintzberg suggested de-emphasizing the manager as a formal decision-maker and proposed instead that the emphasis should be placed on the kinds of roles a manager performs – known as *role theory*. He observed ten key managerial roles that ranged from formal authority to relationships with people (Figure 2.2).

The *interpersonal roles* managers perform are based on the use of formal authority. Mintzberg identifies three types of interpersonal role:

*   *Figurehead* – involving attending ceremonies, addressing the media or taking people to dinner;
*   *Leader* – involving hiring, training and motivating employees, and setting an example for others to follow;
*   *Liaison* – involving dealing with people outside the organization, such as key partners with whom good working relationships are required.

Informational roles flow from the interpersonal roles and are associated with fulfilling the roles of figurehead, leader and/or liaison:

*   *Monitor* – involving seeking information that may be of value;
*   *Disseminator* – involving knowledge transfer between staff in the workplace;
*   *Spokesman* – in dealing with external clients, professionals and interested parties.

The informational roles lead naturally to a range of *decisional roles*:

• *Entrepreneur* – the initiator of change, often taking risks;
• *Disturbance handler* – dealing with disputes and strikes;
• *Resource allocator* – deciding who will be allocated resources;
• *Negotiator* – involving negotiation on behalf of the organization both internally (to staff groups and unions) or externally (to suppliers, clients, governments and so on).

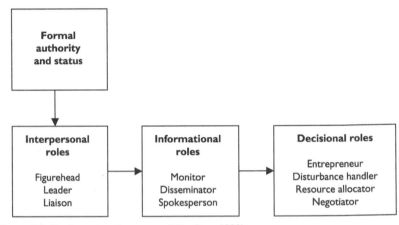

Figure 2.2 Ten key roles of managers (Mintzberg 1989)

Why do organizations need managers?

Following on from his analysis of the ten key roles of a manager, Mintzberg concluded that organizations needed managers for a range of key reasons:

• to ensure the organization serves its purpose and is efficient in the production of goods or services;
• to design and maintain the stability of the operations of the organization;
• to take charge of strategy-making and ensure the organization can adapt to its environment;
• to ensure the organization meets the ends of its bosses and clients;
• to serve as the informational link between the organization and the outside world; and
• to act as a formal authority in operating the organization's 'status system'.

Studies of managerial work such as Mintzberg's role theory have improved understanding of what managers *really* do. You will realize now that managers fulfil many different roles in the course of their work, and identifying these roles should give you a greater appreciation of the management process. However, much management theory tends to be based on the private sector, as well as in the context of high-income countries. So what evidence is there that these principles hold true in public sector health care organizations or in low-income countries with different cultures and contexts?

Management in health care organizations

Activity 2.2

1 What do you think are the key differences between management of a manufacturing industry in the private sector and those in a health care organization in the public sector?
2 What key similarities of management apply to both?

Feedback

1 There are many differences that you may have highlighted. A public sector health care organization has:

- the aim of providing a service, or for promoting health, rather than for making a profit – the public sector ethos;
- a greater role for managers in managing people, especially of professionals who may hold considerable power and status;
- a socio-political environment, since health care is often subject to political debate, public accountability, media scrutiny and top-down reform;
- a higher level of legislation, governance and statutory control;
- a tendency for more rigid personnel policies, fixed salary gradings, career structures and procedures for both promotion and dismissal;
- a greater level of bureaucracy and unionization.

2 Despite these differences, Mullins argues that there are at least four key similarities, or basic principles, that adhere to both:

- the efficiency and effectiveness of their operation;
- the clarification of aims and objectives;
- the design of a suitable structure;
- carrying out essential administrative functions.

A key debate in public sector management in recent years has been the appropriateness of adopting private management practices – so called 'new public management' or the 'new managerialism'. In many countries, the adoption of private sector techniques in public services has become commonplace. For example, in the UK, the adoption of 'general management' into the NHS in the late 1980s, the process of privatization and contracting-out, and the adoption of an internal market in health care have all been attempts to adopt private sector strategies. Their impact, however, has generally been regarded as sub-optimal since a public sector manager's resource decisions are heavily regulated, there is little competition within the system, there is no overall profit or loss measure of efficiency, and processes are heavily influenced by policy boundaries that constrain managerial freedoms.

Management in low- and middle-income countries

The study of management and managerial work has too often been confined to high-income countries with strong market economies. There are cultural differences in low-income countries that may have an influence on managerial work and its meaning. Blunt and Jones (1992), for example, show that studies comparing managerial behaviour between Chinese, African and Western managers differed greatly in the nature and extent of the social welfare for employees and in the variety and depth of personnel issues which found their way to senior managers. As an illustration, they quote a case described by Boisot and Guoling (1988) of a recently retired Chinese worker who had been with a firm for many years but now was bored with sitting at home all day. He walked into the director's office begging for a full-time job – the matter being dealt with personally by the director. Moreover, there was a higher degree of 'centralization' of decision-making, reflecting a cultural wish to keep a close eye on the goings on in the organization. Vengroff et al. (1991) observed that public sector managers in Africa tended to adhere far more to text-book (rules and regulations) approaches to managerial decision-making than Western managers, who were less structured. Blunt and Jones (1992) conclude that institutional and cultural contexts mean managers in low-income countries tend to be more restrained and considered in their actions.

It is clear from studies in high-, middle- and low-income countries that managerial behaviour varies according to a range of environmental, cultural, political and demographic factors. For example, a major study of 1868 'management events' undertaken across nine countries in southern Africa (Angola, Botswana, Lesotho, Malawi, Mozambique, Swaziland, Tanzania, Zambia and Zimbabwe) examined five 'common complaints' about public sector administrators (Montgomery, 1987):

- that they operate in personal fiefdoms because the notion of a service to the public is much less of an incentive than their economic responsibilities to their immediate and extended families;
- that managers are too concerned with operational issues ('fire-fighting'), 'territory' and status, than with policy and strategy;
- that (party) politics and ideological rhetoric interfere with the functioning and effectiveness of organizations;
- that high-performing managers are more likely to be found in the private sector; and
- that organizations and managers are resistant to change.

Montgomery found some truth in all these allegations, especially the importance given to rules and procedures, though the statements were clearly also oversimplifications. Blunt and Jones' (1992) observation was that managers needed to be given the training and ability to take more risks, be more experimental and outward-looking, and more client-oriented, yet were unlikely to be given such opportunities due to political upheavals and opposition to decentralization. Whether these conclusions are really any different from experiences in high-income countries is a matter of debate. If you imagine a group of doctors within a large general hospital and replaced the word 'families' with 'professional elites', then arguably you might find that all five points are just as relevant!

Summary

Managers have many different roles and management has many elements within it. Management is primarily an activity that coordinates and influences people towards a set of organizational objectives. There are important differences in the role and function of managers in health care organizations in the public sector compared to private sector industries, and managerial behaviour varies according to a range of environmental, cultural, political and demographic factors. However, all organizations face similar challenges and in the next chapter you will consider the generic managerial skills and competencies required to undertake managerial tasks effectively.

References

Blunt, P. and Jones, M. (1992) *Managing Organisations in Africa*. New York: De Gruyter.

Boisot, M. and Guoliang, X. (1988) The nature of managerial work – Chinese style?, paper presented to the International Conference on Management in China Today, Leuven, Belgium, 19–21 June, quoted in P. Blunt and M. Jones (1992) *Managing Organisations in Africa*. New York: De Gruyter.

Brech, E. (1975) *Principles and Practice of Management*, 3rd edn. London: Longman.

Dale, E. (1965) *Management: Theory and Practice*. New York: McGraw-Hill.

Drucker, P. (1977) *Management*. London: Pan Books.

Fayol, H. (1949) *General and Industrial Management*. New York: Pitman.

Mintzberg, H. (1989) *Mintzberg on Management*. New York: Free Press.

Montgomery, J. (1987) Probing managerial behaviour: image and reality in Southern Africa', *World Development*, 15(7): 911–29.

Mullins, L.J. (1999) *Management and Organizational Behaviour*, 5th edn. London: *Financial Times* and Pitman Publishing.

Taylor, F.W. (1911) *The Principles of Scientific Management*. New York: Harper Row.

Vengroff, R., Belhaj, M. and Ndiaye, M. (1991) The nature of managerial work in the public sector: an African perspective, *Public Administration and Development*, 7: 273–88.

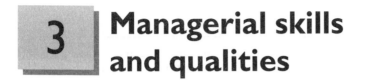

3 Managerial skills and qualities

Overview

To manage effectively, managers require a range of competencies ranging from technical competence, conceptual ability (vision), and relational and social skills. This chapter builds a picture of the core qualities required of a manager in health services by the 'level' at which he or she works. The chapter concludes with an examination of how managerial roles in health care are changing in many countries and the potential new roles that may be required.

Learning objectives

After working through this chapter you will be able to:

- **recognize the different types of skills required of managers in health services;**
- **understand how managers at different levels of an organization require different skills;**
- **understand the qualities of effective managers and the notion of 'managerial competence';**
- **suggest ways in which the future management of health services will require new managerial roles to be developed.**

Key terms

Conceptual skill The ability of managers to understand the complexities and issues within an organization and the role and strength of management within it.

Human skill The ability of managers to work with and through people, including the abilities to lead and to motivate.

Managerial competencies These are specifically developed criteria based on the key managerial skills (technical, human and conceptual) required for a particular job.

Technical skill The ability of a manager to use knowledge, methods, techniques and equipment necessary for the performance of a specific task.

Managerial skills

In the previous chapter the tasks and key roles of a manager were detailed. You will have learned from this that a manager's role in a health care organization is as much in developing the art of human relationships as it is in the technical aspects of what constitutes the most effective management. Management skills refer to the competencies a manager holds to undertake these roles effectively. First classified by Katz (1955) and subsequently adopted by others, such as Hersey and Blanchard (1988), there are three general categories of skills that managers must possess:

1 *Technical skills* – the ability of the manager to use knowledge, methods, techniques and equipment necessary for the performance of a specific task. Such skills can be acquired through training, education and work experience.
2 *Human skills* – the ability of managers to work with and through people, including the abilities to lead and to motivate.
3 *Conceptual skills* – the ability of managers to understand the complexities and issues within an organization and the role and strength of management within it. Conceptual skills are particularly important to enable managers to act according to the goals of the organization as whole, rather than to a specific department.

Activity 3.1

Suppose that Gloria, a nurse leader, has the goal of improving the quality of nursing care amongst a team of eight nurses within a hospital unit specializing in the treatment of HIV/AIDS and STDs. Which of the above three skills would she most need to achieve her objective?

Feedback

All three skills will be essential to Gloria in improving the quality of care that her team of nurses provide. She needs to have technical skills to understand and demonstrate the way comprehensive and individualized nursing care needs to be delivered to patients with HIV/AIDS, so showing her nurse team exactly what is expected through expert teaching and perhaps some work-based training. Gloria also needs considerable human, or social, skills, to ensure that nurses remain empowered and motivated to do their jobs. Her skill as a role model may be especially important in accomplishing this task. Finally, she also needs conceptual skills to understand how the development of a better nursing service will impact on the effectiveness of the health care facility as a whole (adapted from La Monica, 1994).

Management skills by levels of management

Managers at different levels of an organizational hierarchy require different amounts of technical, human and conceptual skills. Hence, staff who are directly supervised by senior managers and who have little devolved management responsibility tend to undertake technical activities, whilst senior staff with wider strategic responsibilities need to be more conceptually aware. This association is illustrated in Figure 3.1. Note how human skills are a constant at all levels and occupy the greater part of the management function. This reflects the arguments from Chapter 2 that showed how much greater the time spent by managers was on relational rather than technical management issues.

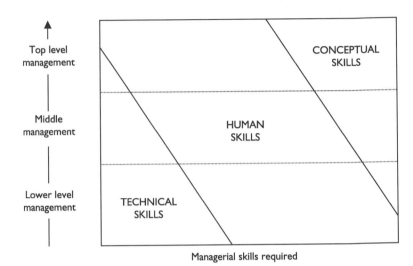

Figure 3.1 Management skills by levels of management (Katz 1955)

Figure 3.1 may seem a simplistic association but having the correct blend of skills for the job at each level is important. For example, it is clearly not necessary that a chief executive should have to understand the technicalities of epidemiology and the process of health needs assessment (though its purpose and meaning should be understood in order to interpret the results and inform an effective strategic response as a result). Similarly, highly trained managerial leaders probably ought not to be stuck doing technical tasks, such as inputting data or undertaking patient surveys.

Managerial competencies

In progressive health care organizations, newly appointed managers with specific technical expertise are often enrolled in training and development programmes such that they might develop their *managerial competencies* and progress up the management hierarchy. Managerial competencies are specifically developed criteria based on key qualities (technical, human and conceptual) for a specific job. In health care management, and the public sector more generally, such competencies are often compared to national standards allowing the skills and progress of a manager to be assessed. Chapters 10 and 11 examine performance management techniques in more detail.

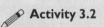 **Activity 3.2**

If you are a manager, do you think you could improve in your role? Do you think those managers you know best have all the necessary qualities that are needed to fulfil their roles effectively?

Feedback

The chances are, if you are being truly honest with yourself and with others, the answer is probably not. This is because managers rarely achieve the status of being super-competent in their jobs since they have either reached their level of competence or been promoted above it, to higher positions. The lack of highly competent managers in health care, or indeed any other organization, is not surprising given the range of qualities (or competencies) that are needed at every level. But that does not mean that a manager should not seek continually to improve.

Activity 3.3

Based on what you have learnt from the first three chapters of this book:

1 Think of a manager you know well and write the name of his role at the top of Table 3.1 (for the sake of anonymity in this analysis, the manager will be called Nick). Then, in the first column, construct a list of ten key qualities that you would assign to the most competent or successful person filling that role.

Table 3.1 Nick's managerial competency analysis table

Management role:

Write down in the space below ten key qualities required for Nick to be 'super-competent' at this job	Note here your assessment of Nick's level of competence to each quality indicator
1	
2	
3	
4	
5	
6	
7	
8	
9	
10	

What are Nick's three key development needs as a manager?

1

2

3

What actions would you recommend to Nick to improve his competencies?

2 Make an honest analysis, using your own personal opinion, of Nick's ability to fulfil the qualities you have created. Note down if Nick is 'super-competent', 'highly competent', 'competent' or 'not competent' in these different tasks.

3 What does the comparison of 'ideal' qualities and 'actual' qualities tell you about Nick's development needs as a manager?

4 What key skills need to be developed for Nick to improve his competencies, and how would you address those needs if you were Nick's mentor in the organization?

Feedback

1 The list of qualities needed to manage to the best effect will vary by the type and role of the manager you have chosen to assess. From your reading, you may have divided the skills needed across the three themes of technical expertise, social skills and conceptual ability. However, it may have become clear to you that actually many of the core competencies for the role interconnect and overlap between these fields. You might like to compare your list with the eleven qualities for successful managers derived from work into the nature of management by Pedler et al. (1994) that is illustrated in Figure 3.2.

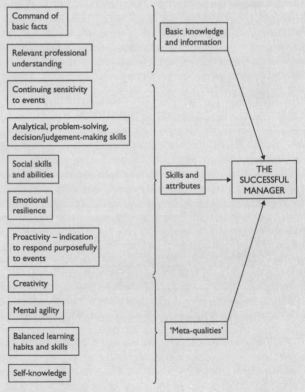

Figure 3.2 The qualities of a successful manager

Notice that each individual quality in their analysis can be placed under the three key headings of technical (basic knowledge and information), human (skills and attributes) and conceptual skills ('meta-qualities').

2, 3 Your analysis of Nick's competencies, compared to the 'ideal' set, may be biased to your own opinions but you should have discovered certain strengths and weaknesses in Nick's capabilities. For example, you may have found him to be strong in technical and human skills but weaker conceptually.

4 Your plan for Nick's development should have concentrated on developing his weaker skills. Possible approaches may have involved education and training, mentorship, and the use of a competency framework as a tool for self-improvement.

The scope and role of what managers do in health care organizations has developed over time. In many high-income countries the devolution of resources and power to front-line professionals has created a new cadre of managers amongst such groups. Moreover, the replacement of monolithic 'command and control' health care organizations in favour of networks of semi-autonomous and even private professionally led organizations has been commonplace. As a result, in many countries, managers of health services have a far wider remit than simply assigning tasks or dictating responsibilities to others and need to embrace more fully their roles as leaders, motivators, change agents and team builders.

Summary

In order to undertake a management task effectively, a combination of technical, human and conceptual skills are required. The mix of skills required differ depending at what level of seniority the manager works. As they progress, managers need to improve their skills and the use of managerial competencies can be helpful in determining key areas for self-improvement and for assessing progress.

References

Hersey, P. and Blanchard, K. (1988) *Management of Organizational Behaviour: Utilizing Human Resources*, 5th edn. New York: Prentice Hall.

Katz, R. (1955) Skills of an effective administrator, *Harvard Business Review*, 33: 33–42.

La Monica, E. (1994) *Management in Health Care: A Theoretical and Experiential Approach*. Basingstoke: Palgrave-Macmillan.

Mullins, L.J. (1999) *Management and Organizational Behaviour*, 5th edn. London: Financial Times and Pitman Publishing.

Pedler, M., Burgoyne, J. and Boydell, T. (1994) *A Manager's Guide to Self Development*, 3rd edn. New York: McGraw-Hill.

4 Problem solving

Overview

The roles and skills of managers that you learnt about in the last two chapters might be viewed as prerequisites for achieving organizational goals. This chapter examines how accomplishing goals requires a conscious, identifiable strategy – a framework known as the 'problem-solving method'. The first part of this chapter examines the theoretical process of problem solving and the second employs a case study to examine how you might adopt such methods in the context of health services management.

Learning objectives

After working through this chapter you will be able to:

- **give reasons for the shift away from classical management towards the contingency approach;**
- **understand the process of 'problem solving' and why this is important in the practice of management;**
- **understand how to apply the problem-solving method.**

Key terms

Contingency approaches Theories which suggest that different behaviours are required in different situations and that successful leaders are those who can move flexibly from one style to another as the situation changes.

Problem-solving method A framework upon which all management practices are built, consisting of problem identification, problem definition, problem analysis, developing solutions, and recommending actions.

Classical management theory and the contingency approach

As you learnt in Chapter 2, classical management thinking in the early twentieth century was dominated by the search for a 'one best way' to do things through single, universal solutions to management problems. However, it was soon realized that finding appropriate managerial solutions in any specific case was dependent on context and interrelated elements – or contingencies. The *contingency approach*, therefore, refers to the view that managerial solutions need to be case-specific in order to develop the best managerial response to perceived problems (Buchanan and Huczynski, 1997).

The problem-solving method

The problem-solving method, developed by La Monica (1994), is one of a number of frameworks that have been developed to help managers respond to contingencies. It has particular relevance to managers in health services since the roots of the framework were developed through an analysis of the nursing process and how problems in providing nursing care were found and resolved (La Monica, 1985).

Problem identification

The first step is problem identification. A problem is identified when the actual situation significantly differs from the optimal situation. To determine a problem area, the manager needs to gather, examine and interpret information and then decide if the problem is important enough to warrant attention.

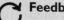 **Activity 4.1**

What sources of information do you think a manager needs to be able to identify problems effectively?

Feedback

Key sources of information might include clinicians, superiors, managerial colleagues and patients. Your own point of view is also important, as is your awareness of the perceptions of others. Holding team meetings or focus groups can often be a good way of identifying and defining problems.

Problem definition

Having determined that a problem exists, the next step is to define the problem by understanding its nature. For example, if you identified that the performance of a clinical team was a problem, you would need to understand all the aspects of what contributes to their overall performance to find out where the problem lies. For example, is it because they are communicating poorly with each other, or do they lack some key information or guidance?

A clearly defined problem is essential in order to mobilize efforts to address it. Moreover, it may be that the problem has several steps. For example, if the optimal goal is to provide best care for an older person with complex needs, the problem might first require a short-term solution such as writing an appropriate care plan.

In defining the problem in relation to the ultimate goal, you will probably find that there is a series of interrelated problems that need to be addressed in a step-by-step fashion.

Problem analysis

Having identified the boundaries of a problem, the next step is to analyse the problem. At this stage you need to ask yourself four key questions:

1 Why does the problem exist?
2 Which staff groups need to be involved in order for the problem to be fixed?
3 Is the group able to respond to the problem that is presented to them?
4 What managerial tactics should be employed to meet the group's need in addressing the problem?

The purpose of these questions is to broaden a manager's understanding of the problem.

Developing solutions

The next step is to develop solutions for achieving the key goal. This might be done through an unstructured process of brainstorming or creative thinking with colleagues to develop a range of options. The process might also be more structured using a range of diagnostic assessment tools (which you will learn about in Chapters 17 and 18). Having developed a range of solutions, the positive and negative elements of each should be discussed with all stakeholders to assess which might enable a problem to be solved and, as a result, for you to move towards the optimal or overall goal.

Recommending actions

Although only one strategy has to be chosen, often there is no single solution likely to meet all of the positive elements and none of the negative ones. Managerial judgement based on the development of a range of options is important before action can be recommended. But this does not always mean that optimal outputs will result. It is because of the contingent nature of management (because organizations and professionals have to adapt continually to meet core goals) that the problem-solving method is a recurrent issue for managers – especially in health services management.

Applying the problem-solving approach: a case study

For the remainder of this chapter you will undertake activities designed to help you apply the different elements of the problem-solving method in practice. The following scenario (adapted from La Monica, 1994) is an example of problems encountered by a nurse manager in an orthopaedic unit within a 400-bed hospital. As you read it, imagine that you are the nurse manager and think about the problems you have encountered and the potential solutions to the problems you might try to initiate.

The problems of a nurse manager

You are the head nurse of a 48-bed ward for care of the elderly within a 400-bed general hospital. You have been in the position for over seven years and have taken over the management responsibility for the team of nurses working on the ward. Most of the patients require a stay of over two weeks, having either suffered severe trauma or requiring intensive care due to a chronic illness. Some patients, about 20 per cent, need only a short stay (one or two days).

The ward, and the hospital, has a good reputation for quality. The hospital's senior management team, as part of a wider strategy for better patient-based care, have asked you to develop in your ward individualized care plans for patients. However, this policy runs against the traditional (bureaucratic) way things have been run for many years.

Your ward has traditionally practised 'team nursing' in which tasks have been divided into a package of procedures characterized by the use of flow charts, treatment protocols and well-documented routines. Care plans have traditionally been developed on a generic basis for all patients, with nurses checking the protocols within them to see what forms of medication or care are required. Since the tasks are sometimes perceived as boring and repetitive, you have developed a weekly schedule of rotation of tasks.

There are three teams in your ward, each providing good-quality care for one-third of the patients. Each team has a complement of different nurse skills and physiotherapists. Turnover of staff has been fairly low and the individuals in the team have developed good working relationships. Given their high standard of care and experience, you have generally allowed the nurse teams to work independently, and your other duties mean you cannot see them every day.

In the three weeks since the documentation about introducing patient-based care and the need to develop individual care plans in consultation with patients was distributed, you have noticed a change in attitude amongst the teams. Nurses have increasingly been late in their reporting procedures and seem more interested in their own speciality rather than working for the team. Though patients seem happy, complaints have been rising amongst the nurses and arguments between staff have been occurring. Individualized care plans have been completed, but there seems to have been little real change in the way nurses operate at the bedside, where nurse time has actually decreased.

✎ Activity 4.2

What is the key problem that is identifiable in this case?

Feedback

The process you should have followed was to first write down the key problem areas based on the differences between the optimal scenario (the goal) and the actual scenario (the present situation). You may have identified the problems shown in Table 4.1:

Table 4.1 Identifying the problem

Problem	Optimal	Actual
Team working	Good team working	Less team working and increase in arguments
Lateness	No lateness	Lateness is increasing
Routine nursing care	Nursing care becomes more individualized and client-based	Nursing care is actually less individualized
Time spent with patients	Increasing	Decreasing

Source: Adapted from La Monica (1994)

Activity 4.3

How would you define and describe these problems?

Feedback

The four problems are clearly related to the central problem that nursing care has become repetitive and monotonous, with staff lacking motivation and little opportunity to develop new skills. The nurse manager's key goal, however, is to ensure that patients have input and ownership of their care plans – not motivating staff *per se*. In developing a specific statement to describe the problem, you might have developed something like the following:

Optimal – the patients and nurse team leaders develop individualized care plans.
Actual – the patient has no input into the nursing care plan.
Problem – routine nursing care is not individualized.
Goal – to individualize nursing care plans by motivating the nursing team to build in patients' views.

Activity 4.4

What tactics might you employ to address the problem in your role as nurse manager?

○ Feedback

In analysing the problem, you may have considered a number of strategies which you as the nurse manager could adopt to fit the context of the problem. By looking, or gaining information, on the motivations of yourself and the nursing staff, you might have developed the following synthesis:

Yourself (nurse manager) – you enjoy working with the nursing team and are committed to solving the problem.

Your nurse team – since the team has been together for some time, it is likely that they remain committed to a high quality of patient care. Their lack of motivation, therefore, was probably more to do with an unwillingness to move from an established model of care to a new model, since planning nursing care with the patient had never been a part of nursing practice in the past.

Key tactics – a conscious effort is required on behalf of the nurse manager to get nurses to implement the new approach whilst acknowledging they may feel uncomfortable with the new processes. A high task, high relationship approach is needed – defining what nurses need to do but discussing issues and feelings openly to avoid bad feeling amongst the nurse team of having the system imposed upon them. This is a form of managing change that you will examine further in Chapters 18 and 19.

✎ Activity 4.5

What other potential actions might you propose?

○ Feedback

You may have considered many, but you should have analysed the positive and negative aspects of the process. For example, you might have thought of three options:

- Hold regular social events to increase team morale and to discuss the development of individualized care plans on an informal basis. The potential positives are the development of a network of informational exchange and the greater ability to air grievances and problems leading to more openness. The potential negatives are the continued lack of direction at a systemic level, the fact that not all staff will attend and that the process may be trivialized.
- Hold a meeting with nurse team leaders to discuss how to achieve the goal of developing individualized care plans. The potential positives are as above, with the additional possibility of arriving at a joint plan of action. The potential disadvantage is that nurse opposition might result in a stand-off of views.
- Arrange a meeting between senior managers in the hospital (keen to see patient-based care advanced as a hospital strategy) to discuss their approach with the nursing team. The potential positive might be motivational – the feeling of high-level support for the nurses and an explanation of the hospital's patient-based mission. A potential negative might be the opposite – resentment that senior managers were not aware of the nursing team's concerns before the patient-based initiative was imposed.

Activity 4.6

Based on the three possible actions given above, which would you recommend?

Feedback

All three have merits and potential problems. Given that the team has been mature and cohesive in the past, and you as team leader seemingly retain respect, the second option might be most appropriate since the nurse team requires direction and motivation but also a formal forum to air their fears and grievances. Whichever option you chose, the underlying criterion is the ability to neutralize the effects of negative outcomes.

The implementation of your remedial action needs to be evaluated to understand whether it has achieved its desired consequences. It is likely that the solution, or action plan, that you develop will only be one part of a wider strategy to implement patient-based care in your part of the hospital.

Summary

Problem solving is a key managerial task. In this chapter you have learned about the problem-solving method and used a case study through which to understand the ways in which it can be applied. It has shown how a manager needs to take a carefully crafted approach to the management of problems from their diagnosis to implementation and evaluation.

References

Buchanan, D. and Huczynski, A. (1997) *Organizational Behaviour: An Introductory Text*, 3rd edn. London: Prentice Hall.

La Monica, E. (1985) *The Humanistic Nursing Process*. Boston: Jones and Bartlett.

La Monica, E. (1994) *Management in Health Care: A Theoretical and Experiential Approach*. Basingstoke: Palgrave-Macmillan.

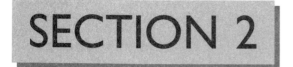

SECTION 2

Health care funding

5 | Funding health care systems

Overview

Management textbooks often tend to examine the functions involved in managing people and managing change but miss out the implications for managers of the way health services are financed and purchased. This chapter, the first of three on this subject, reviews the key functions involved in funding health care and the different financial mechanisms used. This chapter concentrates on how revenue is collected (for example, via general taxation, social insurance, private insurance and direct payments), how funds are pooled, and how care is then purchased from providers.

Learning objectives

After working through this chapter you will be able to:

- **understand the three key functions involved in funding health systems;**
- **distinguish between the ways different countries finance health services;**
- **recognize the advantages and disadvantages of different financing methods.**

Key terms

Community financing Collective action of local communities to finance health services through pooling out-of-pocket payments and ensuring services are accountable to the community.

Loans (grants, donations) External aid used to fund services, usually with a set of conditions attached.

Out-of-pocket (direct) payments Payment made by a patient to a provider.

Private health insurance Voluntary insurance to cover health care costs based on the individual's level of risk.

Purchasing The process by which funds are used to pay providers.

Revenue collection The process by which a health system receives money.

Risk pooling A way in which revenue is managed to ensure that the risk of having to pay for health care is borne by all rather than by the individual.

Social health insurance Compulsory contributions to a health insurance fund gaining individual or group entitlement to health care benefits – usually based on employer and employee contributions.

Taxation An method of financing health care and other public services based on either a direct payroll or income tax or indirect taxes on goods and services.

Managing the funding system

Health care funding is a key part of the interaction between providers, managers and citizens. The main managerial challenge is to ensure the necessary technical, organizational and institutional arrangements so that providers will be motivated to increase health and improve the responsiveness of the system to health care needs. There are three key functions to a funding system:

1 *Revenue collection* – the process by which a health system receives money.
2 *Pooling resources* – how revenue is managed to ensure that the risk of having to pay for health care is borne by all members of the pool rather than by each contributor individually.
3 *Purchasing care* – the process by which pooled funds are used to pay providers in order to deliver a set of health care interventions.

There are different ways that these three functions are performed. They may be highly integrated in a single organization (such as in a 'managed care' system like Kaiser Permanente in the USA) or they may be separate tasks – for example, one organization may collect and pool funds (for example, a government) whilst others may purchase services (such as a health authority) and still others provide the care (pharmacies, primary care practices, hospitals and so on) (Kutzin, 2001). This chapter will assess how each of these functions can be performed.

Revenue collection: an introduction

✏️ Activity 5.1

There are three key concerns in revenue collection. Thinking first about your own country and second about the world as a whole:

1 Who pays? What are the sources from which funds are taken?
2 What is the type of payment? How are contributions made?
3 Who collects it? Which agencies are involved in the process?

↻ **Feedback**

Compare the range of funding sources, types of payment and collection methods that you thought of with those summarized in Table 5.1.

Table 5.1 Methods of revenue collection

Who pays? What are the 'sources' from which funds are taken?	• Individuals • Households • Employees • Employers – firms and corporate bodies • Foreign governments • NGOs and charities
How are contributions made? What is the 'type' of payment?	• Direct and indirect taxes • Compulsory insurance contributions and payroll taxes • Voluntary insurance premiums • Medical savings accounts • Out-of-pocket payments • Loans, grants and donations
Who collects the revenue? Which agencies can be involved in this process?	• Government agencies – central, regional and local • Independent public body or social security agency (insurance agent) • Community health insurance fund • Private 'not-for-profit' insurance fund • Private 'for-profit' insurance fund • Direct to providers

Source: Adapted from Mossialos et al. (2002).

1 You can see that there are several sources and ways that revenue can be collected. Funds derive primarily from the population (individuals and/or those that employ them).

2 Funding mechanisms include general taxation, mandated social insurance contributions (usually salary-related), voluntary private insurance contributions (usually risk-related), out-of-pocket payments and donations. Most high-income countries use taxation and social health insurance. By contrast, low-income countries depend far more on out-of-pocket financing and donor contributions.

3 Collection agents vary from public to private not-for-profit and private for-profit as well as direct fees paid directly to providers.

Figure 5.1 illustrates how the diversity of the different funding sources, collection methods and collection agents interrelate.

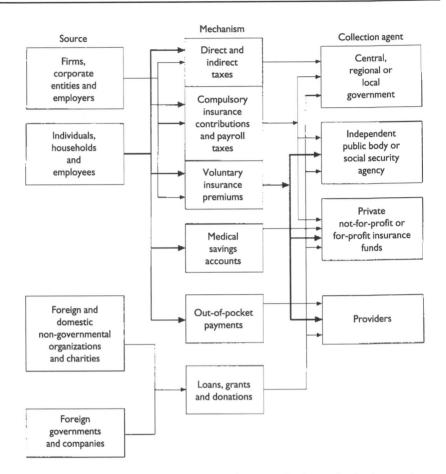

Figure 5.1 Examples of funding sources, contribution mechanisms and collection agents (Mossialos et al. 2002)

✎ Activity 5.2

The following multiple choice quiz gives you an opportunity to reflect on the diversity of revenue collection methods. Spend only a few minutes and make guesses if necessary – it is a test designed to show you the diversity of revenue collection arrangements rather than a direct test of your knowledge.

1   Match the following countries with their *primary* source of health care finance:

(a) USA   (i)   Social insurance
(b) UK   (ii)   Local and general taxation
(c) Germany   (iii) General taxation
(d) Sweden   (iv)   Out-of-pocket payments
(e) Bangladesh   (v)   Private health insurance

2 Match the following regions to a description of their key funding arrangements.

(a) Latin America
(b) Sub-Saharan Africa
(c) Eastern Europe (before 1989)
(d) USA

(i) Taxation, community financing and out-of-pocket payments
(ii) Mixed model of social health insurance, private health insurance and taxation for public health
(iii) Private health insurance and social health insurance for the elderly, disabled and the poor
(iv) Taxation

Feedback

1 (a) (v); (b) (iii); (c) (i); (d) (ii); (e) (iv)

2 (a) (ii); (b) (i); (c) (iv); (d) (iii)

Activity 5.3

Look at Figures 5.2 and 5.3 which examine the differences between some European countries on the proportion of total health care expenditure derived from social health insurance and from taxation.

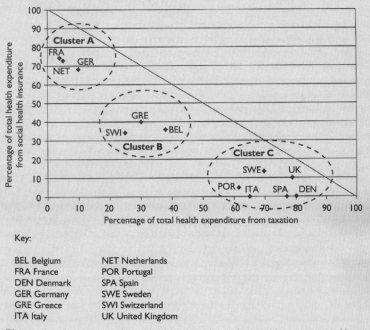

Key:

BEL Belgium
FRA France
DEN Denmark
GER Germany
GRE Greece
ITA Italy

NET Netherlands
POR Portugal
SPA Spain
SWE Sweden
SWI Switzerland
UK United Kingdom

Figure 5.2 Percentage of total health expenditure financed by taxation and by social health insurance in selected Western European countries in 1998 (Mossialos et al. 2002)

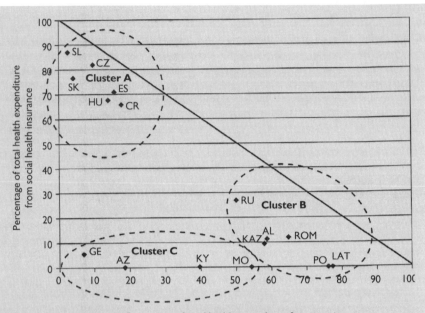

Percentage of total health expenditure from taxation

Key:

AL Albania	KY Kyrgyzstan
AZ Azerbaijan	LAT Latvia
CR Croatia	MO Republic of Moldova
CZ Czech Republic	PO Poland
ES Estonia	ROM Romania
GE Georgia	RU Russia
HU Hungary	SK Slovakia
KAZ Kazakhstan	SL Slovenia

Figure 5.3 Percentage of total health expenditure financed by taxation and by social health insurance in sixteen countries in Central and Eastern Europe and the former Soviet Union, 1997 (Mossialos et al. 2002)

1 What is the significance of countries in Cluster A, B and C?
2 Name five countries whose predominant source of revenue is social health insurance.
3 Name five countries whose predominant source of revenue is taxation.
4 Why is it that no country has 100 per cent of its spending covered from a combination of taxation and social insurance? What other funding sources do you think make up the difference?
5 From Figure 5.3, what do you think has happened to those countries in Cluster C?

Revenue collection: a comparative analysis

According to the World Health Organization (2000), the relative performance of health care systems reflects differences in the ways revenue is collected and administered. The following analysis undertakes a comparative analysis of the advantages and disadvantages of the following different revenue collection methods: taxation, social health insurance, private health insurance, out-of-pocket payments, and loans and donations. It is based on the summary of advantages and disadvantages of funding methods described by Mossialos and colleagues (2002). For each revenue collection method you will be provided with a short overview of the approach before being given the task of assessing its strengths and weaknesses.

Taxation

Taxation methods vary enormously. First, taxes may be raised for unspecified, general purposes or specifically for health (hypothecated). Second, taxes may be direct or indirect. Direct taxes are levied on individuals, households or firms and include mechanisms such as a personal income tax, property tax and company tax. Indirect taxes are taxes on transactions and commodities rather than people, for example a tax on the sales of goods, or export and import taxes. Third, taxes may be raised by central government or locally and used to finance health care in that specific region or locality.

✎ Activity 5.4

What do you think are the main advantages and disadvantages of these different forms of taxation? Write down at least one advantage and one disadvantage for:

1 general versus hypothecated
2 direct versus indirect
3 central versus local government.

↻ **Feedback**

1. Hypothecated taxes have several advantages over general taxes since it links tax and spending directly making it highly transparent where tax money is being spent. However, it reduces the ability to be flexible – investing more resources where needed in an emergency, or taking resources out as a trade-off to another area of expenditure. General taxation also enables tax to be drawn from a far wider variety of sources.

2. Direct taxes, based on incomes, have the advantage of being *progressive*, since high earners contribute more than low earners and the wealth is then redistributed in the form of health benefits for all. In high-income countries the process is administratively simple to collect as there is capacity and ability to do so (for example, in a payroll tax). In low-income countries the tax-based option can be logistically unfeasible. Indirect taxes have the disadvantage of being *regressive*, since they do not differentiate payments by income levels. Many indirect taxes are fixed amounts (for example, for a vehicle licence). However, taxation on goods that are regarded to do harm to health – such as tobacco products or alcohol – may deter consumption and help improve health.

3. Local taxes may have certain advantages over a national system, including:

  • greater transparency, since health care expenditure in a local tax system often forms the largest percentage of what a local authority spends (up to 70 per cent in Sweden, for example);
  • improved accountability, as local politicians are closer to their electorate;
  • better responsiveness, to local needs and demands; and
  • the separation of health budgets from competing national demands.

However, it is possible that local taxation leads to differential funding between less and more affluent regions resulting in inequalities in health care provision and the inability to redistribute resources. National taxation avoids these issues, though the process means expenditure on health has to compete with other demands, such as defence, or handed away through tax cuts.

Social health insurance

Social health insurance contributions are usually compulsory and shared between employee and the employer. The collection agent can vary from a single national insurance fund (such as in Croatia and Slovakia) or devolved to local branches of a national fund (as in Romania), to smaller independent funds (as in France), or through individual health funds either by occupation or by geographical area (as in Germany).

Like taxation-based funding, a key advantage is the ability to create a large risk pool through the prepayment of funds. Moreover, social health insurance funds are often more socially acceptable to the public (especially where there is some mistrust of the state) because budgetary and spending decisions on health care become ring-fenced and are somewhat protected from political interference.

Key disadvantages include:

  • Employers are often asked to pay a contribution, thus increasing labour costs. If social insurance is not mandatory, then this offers a perverse incentive on the part of employers to pay below the minimum threshold, or outsource activities so that the burden falls on contractors or the self-employed. These practices are common in countries with newly established health insurance systems (such as in those countries in Figure 5.3). Employers, faced with an adverse economic climate, have tried to minimize labour costs by evading social health insurance contributions, which in the countries of Cluster C in Figure 5.3 have led to significant problems in the funding system.

- Eligibility in social health insurance systems is based on employment, potentially restricting access to care for the elderly and the unemployed.
- Coverage tends to focus on personal health care rather than on public health and health improvement measures.
- Social health insurance may not cover the costs of provision. Indeed, most social health insurance systems include elements of taxation-based subsidies and/or out-of-pocket co-payments to bridge the gap between income and expenditure and stop the potential fragmentation of coverage.

Private health insurance

Private health insurance has three main forms: substitutive, supplementary and complimentary.

Substitutive insurance is an alternative to social insurance and is often available to sections of the population who may be excluded from public cover or who are free to opt out of the national system. In Germany and the Netherlands, for example, employees earning over a certain income are excluded from coverage in the social insurance scheme (though they still make the payments) and are required to take out private insurance to get the care they require.

Supplementary insurance is an additional payment in order to receive benefits on top of those offered in a social insurance scheme. It may allow quicker access to care, to access better facilities (such as a separate room, rather than being on a general ward) or covers the costs of any co-payments (such as drugs or in-patient stays). In France, for example, about 70 per cent of the population takes out supplementary private insurance. Supplementary insurance can lead to inequities between rich and poor in the use of health care.

Complimentary insurance offers full or partial cover for services that are excluded from the social insurance or tax-based scheme, often known as a 'top-up' policy. Complimentary insurance is least affordable to those on low incomes.

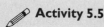 **Activity 5.5**

1 What role does private health insurance play in your country? Is there a significant private insurance market? What proportion of the population subscribe?
2 What are the major disadvantages of private health insurance, compared with taxation and social health insurance?

↻ **Feedback**

1 Unless you live in the USA or Switzerland, private health insurance is likely to be of limited significance in your country. In low-income countries, private insurance accounts for less than 2 per cent of the total and in a high-income country, such as the UK, the figure is only about 12 per cent (Laing and Buisson, 1995). Private health insurance attracts only the most affluent as enrolment is based on the ability to pay.

2 The major disadvantages are:

- *inequity* – of access to care for the poor and elderly who may be those in the population with most need;
- *moral hazard* – neither the consumer nor the provider of care has an incentive to contain costs as the system is fuelled on entitlement to care and reimbursement through a fee-for-service;
- *adverse selection* – where consumers select plans that give them the greatest benefit;
- *cream skimming* – where insurers exclude high-risk and potentially costly insurees;
- *high transaction costs* – related to marketing, administration, claims processing, and handling of reimbursements – in unregulated markets such costs can be very high, for example in the USA they account for about 25–30 per cent of the total;
- *coverage* – economic liberalization policies in many countries, such as Sri Lanka, has seen deregulation and a greater role for private health insurance. However, the approach does not increase coverage of care to the population as a whole.

Out-of-pocket payments

Unlike in the above three *prepayment models*, where it is possible to pool funds and spread risks amongst the population, a health system where individuals have to pay directly, out of their own pockets, for a substantial part of the cost of health services clearly restricts access to those who cannot afford to pay, particularly for expensive care. Most low-income countries, where prepayment systems are unavailable, have introduced some form of out-of-pocket payment in order to raise revenue, recover costs, and improve services (Nolan and Turbat, 1995).

Community financing is a method used in some low-income countries in an attempt to pool funds through out-of-pocket payments. The Bamako Initiative, for example, has been promoted since 1987 in many parts of Africa as a way of promoting access to essential primary care services and drugs by decentralizing health decision-making and revenue collection to local communities (World Bank, 1987). The basis of the approach is to levy a small out-of-pocket payment when a drug is prescribed or care is provided. Having pooled the funds, the local community can then decide how to spend it to meet their needs. Overall, community financing has led to relative improvements in coverage, affordability and utilization of care – but that access from 'marginalized' groups remain unchanged due to the need to pay for care. However, the approach has been successful enough to show that it is possible to raise revenue to cover costs and invest in health services (McPake et al., 1993).

In high-income countries, people are often required to make a personal contribution towards their health care costs (for example, to pay for drugs or to contribute to the cost of visiting a doctor or for staying in a hospital bed). These are known as user fees or co-payments. It is argued that this can contribute to covering health costs and perhaps limit rising demands for care whilst encouraging the use of other facilities. However, it is clear that, depending on the level at which they are set, user fees can dissuade the poor from using services; do not appear to generate adequate revenue to enable sustained improvements to care; and are inequitable (Gilson, 1995).

Loans, grants and donations

In many low-income countries, external aid is a substantial source of funding for the health sector and may account for as much as 90 per cent of the overall health budget (WHO, 1995). External aid takes the form of loans or grants that are usually bound to a set of conditions by the donor. This means that external aid serves not only the recipient's interest but also the donor's political and economic interests too.

The following is a commentary on the use of donations and grants from non-governmental organizations and international banks (WHO, 2000):

Donations and grants to low-income countries

Donor contributions, as a source of revenue for the health system, are of key importance for some developing countries. The absolute amounts of such aid have been large in recent years in Angola, Bangladesh, Ecuador, India, Indonesia, Mozambique, Papua New Guinea, the United Republic of Tanzania and several Eastern European countries, but in the larger countries aid is usually only a small share of total health spending or even of government expenditure. In contrast, several countries, particularly in Africa, depend on donors for a large share of total expenditure on health. The fraction can be as high as 40 per cent (Uganda in 1993) or even 84 per cent (Gambia in 1994) and exceeds 20 per cent in 1996 or 1997 in Eritrea, Kenya, The Lao People's Democratic Republic and Mali. Bolivia, Nicaragua, the United Republic of Tanzania and Zimbabwe have obtained 10 per cent to 20 per cent of their resources for health from donors in one or more recent years.

Most aid comes in the form of projects, which are separately developed and negotiated between each donor and the national authorities. Although by no means unsuccessful, international cooperation through projects can lead to fragmentation and duplication of effort, particularly when many donors are involved, each focusing on their own geographical or programme priorities. Such an approach forces national authorities to devote significant amounts of time and effort to dealing with donors' priorities and procedures, rather than concentrating on strategic stewardship and health programme implementation. Donors and governments are increasingly seeing the need to move away from a project approach towards wider programme support to long-term strategic development that is integrated into the budgetary process of the country. In this respect, sector-wide approaches have been effective in countries such as Bangladesh, Ghana and Pakistan.

✎ **Activity 5.6**

1 Why are low-income countries often reliant on donations and loans?
2 What are the main concerns for a health system that relies on such methods of finance?
3 Give examples of bilateral and multilateral donor agencies.

↻ **Feedback**

1 Donor assistance is very high in many low income countries that do not have the necessary resources or expertise to address health and development needs. In Africa as a whole, for example, 20 per cent of total health care expenditure is provided through loans, grants and donations. Many countries are reliant on such finance for more than 50 per cent of their expenditure.

2 Grants may not increase expenditure in the health sector as governments may use the funds as a substitute for their own expenditure, or they may channel the funds towards other priorities. Donors cannot be relied upon for long-term financial support whilst loans need to be repaid, with interest, imposing a potentially huge burden of debt. Aid and donations, therefore, can do more harm than good if poorly used and administered.

3 Bilateral agencies are donors from a particular country. Examples include USAID and DANIDA, the Danish development agency. Multilateral agencies are funds from a pooled resource between countries. For example, the UNDF (United Nations Development Fund), the World Bank or the European Community.

Pooling resources

Fund pooling is about sharing financial risk between contributors. Prepayment and pooling have significant advantages over out-of-pocket financing for the following reasons:

- economies of scale, allowing for *cross-subsidization* from low- to high-risk people;
- equalization of contributions amongst members, regardless of their risk of needing to use services.

In Table 5.2 you can see that there are several approaches to spreading risk by pooling funds including social health insurance funds, centrally or regionally held budgets as a result of taxation, or smaller community financing pools based on locally agreed contributions. As the examples suggest, a range of agents might collect the money and then contribute to a central pool. There can even be multiple pools with the level of risk-pooling being adjusted to population's risk profile (for example, when resources in a country are devolved to local agencies).

Table 5.2 National examples of approaches to spreading risk and subsidizing the poor

Country	System	Spreading risk	Subsidizing the poor
Colombia	Multiple pools	Competing social security	Organizations, municipal health
Netherlands	Multiple pools: predominantly private competing social insurance organizations	Intra-pool via non-risk-related contribution and inter-pool via central risk equalization fund	Via risk equalization fund, excluding the rich
Republic of Korea	Two main pools: national health insurance and the Ministry of Health National health insurance, however, covers only 30 per cent of total health expenditures of any member	Intra-pool via non-risk-related contribution Explicit single benefit package for all members	Salary-related contribution plus supply-side subsidy via the Ministry of Health and national health insurance from Ministry of Finance allocations Public subsidy for insurance for the poor and farmers
Zambia	Single predominant formal pool: Ministry of Health/Central Board of Health	Intra-pool, implicit single benefit package for all in the Ministry of Health System and at state level Financed via general taxes	Intra-pool via general taxation Supply-side subsidy via the Ministry of Health

Source: World Health Organization (2000)

✎ Activity 5.7

Looking at the four examples of pooling in Table 5.2:

1 Why are large risk pools better than small ones?
2 What are the potential problems facing Colombia with its range of smaller pools?

↻ Feedback

1 Large pools are better than small ones because they can increase resource availability for health services. A large pool has three advantages over small ones:

- economies of scale in administration;
- reduced level of contributions required to protect against uncertain needs;
- ensures that sufficient funds are available to pay for health services.

2 Colombia's fragmented system of small organizations involved in revenue collection and pooling is likely to damage performance of all these three tasks. In Argentina before

1996, there were more than 300 pooling organizations (*Obras Sociales Nacionales*) for workers and their families. Many had fewer than 50,000 members. The administrative capacity and financial reserves required to ensure their financial viability, together with the low wages of their beneficiaries, guaranteed that their health care benefit packages were very limited. In community financing, described in the Bamako initiative, small size and lack of organizational capacity to run them has often threatened their financial sustainability – though the approach is clearly an improvement on individual out-of-pocket payments. Note that it is not the *number* of pools that is the issue here but their size.

Purchasing care

Purchasing is the transfer of pooled resources to service providers on behalf of the population for which the funds were pooled. In most health financing arrangements, pooling and purchasing are integrated within the same organization. However, there have been attempts to decentralize the function by allocating budgets to separate purchasing agents to purchase care (for example, in the UK). Purchasing plays a central role in ensuring coherence of external incentives for providers through contracting, budgeting and payment mechanisms. The process is a key managerial task in health care and is examined in Chapter 6.

The structure of health system financing and provision

You will now appreciate how complex the funding of health services can be and you will appreciate how different countries use a mix of different funding methods. Figure 5.4 provides a comparison of these funding methods across four countries showing the proportionality of the different approaches related to the flow of funds.

Activity 5.8

Thinking of your own country:

1 Fill out the bar chart in Table 5.3 to describe the structure of your country's system of health financing.
2 What do you think are the main policy issues your country needs to address as regards the way health care is financed?

Table 5.3 The structure of your home country's health financing system

Revenue collection	
Pooling	
Purchasing	

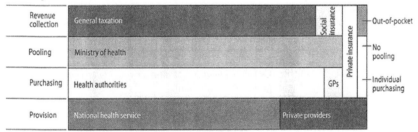

Figure 5.4 Structure of health system financing and provision in four countries

Source: World Health Organization (2000)

↻ **Feedback**

 1 Your chart will be particular to your own country. You might want to check your answer with those involved in the health care system.

 2 Health system policy with regard to collection and pooling resources needs to focus on creating those conditions where the largest possible pool can be created. Where a particular country lacks capacity, and may have a high proportion of care funded from out-of-pocket payments or donors, policy-makers need to promote the development of small pools as a transitional process to developing larger ones. For low-income countries, community financing may be an interim step.

Summary

In this chapter you have examined the three functions by which health care systems are funded: revenue collection, pooling and purchasing. You have seen the complexities of this process and the advantages and disadvantages of the different methods that have been utilized. You have learned that the key elements to stable financing, for the most health care gain to a population, are the ability to prepay for health care and the development of a large enough resource pool to cover risks and to cross-subsidize between low- and high-risk people.

References

Gilson, L. (1995) Management and health care reform in Sub-Saharan Africa, *Social Science and Medicine*, 40(5): 695–710.

Kutzin, A. (2001) A descriptive framework for country-level analysis of health care financing arrangements, *Health Policy*, 56(3): 171–204.

Laing, W. and Buisson, W. (1995) *Laing's Review of Private Health Care*. London: Laing & Buisson.

McPake, B., Hanson, K. and Mills, A. (1993) Community financing of health care in Africa: an evaluation of the Bamako Initiative, *Social Science and Medicine* 36(11): 1383–95.

Mossialos, E., Dixon, A., Figueras, J. and Kutzin, J. (2002) *Funding Health Care: Options for Europe*. Buckingham: Open University Press.

Nolan, B. and Turbat, V. (1995) *Cost Recovery in Public Health Services in Sub-Saharan Africa*. Washington, DC: World Bank.

World Bank (1987) *Financing Health Services in Developing Countries, an Agenda for Reform*. Washington, DC: World Bank.

World Health Organization (1995) *Changes in Sources of Finance*, technical report series 829, Geneva: WHO.

World Health Organization (2000) *The World Health Report 2000. Health Systems: Improving Performance*, Geneva: WHO.

6 Purchasing health services

Overview

From Chapter 5 you will have learned that purchasing health services is the third key function in the funding process. The management of purchasing is essential in ensuring that the providers of services meet the goals of the health system. This chapter examines the three fundamental management challenges to purchasing health services: deciding what to purchase, from whom, and how.

Learning objectives

After working through this chapter you will be able to:

- **understand the importance of strategic purchasing and the financing of essential care packages;**
- **discuss the advantages and disadvantages of different methods of purchasing and understand the incentives on providers contained in each;**
- **understand the internal and external incentives and pressures that funding agencies work with and how these can impact on their ability to perform their functions effectively.**

Key terms

Capitation payments A prospective means of paying health care staff based on the number of people they provide care for.

Diagnosis related group (DRG) Classification system that assigns patients to categories on the basis of the likely cost of their episode of hospital care. Used as basis for determining level of prospective payment by purchaser.

Essential package of care A strategy for purchasing services that achieves the greatest reduction in the burden of disease with available resources.

Fee-for-service A means of paying health care staff on the basis of the actual items of care provided.

Prospective payment Paying providers before any care is delivered, based on predefined activity levels and anticipated costs.

Retrospective payment Paying provides for any work they have undertaken, with no agreement in advance.

Strategic purchasing The identification and procurement of the best care to meet the goals for the health care system.

Purchasing health services

Purchasing health services faces three fundamental challenges:

• which packages of care to buy;
• from whom to buy them;
• how to buy them.

Size is important for purchasing organizations since large purchasers not only have administrative advantages in terms of economies of scale, they also have better bargaining capacity over price and quality. Identifying the best packages of care and the best providers means a manager must either search for the best deals and/or establish strategic alliances with providers to disseminate best practice amongst them and help develop their functions and capacity.

Which packages of care to buy: strategic purchasing

Strategic purchasing requires a continuous search for the best interventions, or care packages, to purchase. There are two levels to this. The first level is related to stewardship – how society or policy-makers determine the goals of the health system and balances equity, efficiency, choice, responsiveness and quality. The second level is the responsibility for the identification of the interventions that will achieve these goals best. The latter implies responsibility for creating incentives and negotiating with providers to achieve this.

Essential care packages

Many countries (in particular low-income countries) are unable to afford to provide health care for the entire population and face major imbalances in resource allocation – for example, between urban and rural regions, and between rich and poor. The ability to define priorities to ensure maximum health gain for the money that is available to purchase health services becomes a key task. A policy of *essential care packages* (ECPs) has been promoted in many such countries to purchase services that have the highest potential for reducing the burden of disease (Bobadilla and Cowley, 1995). The key reasons for introducing ECPs are to:

• provide the most effective care to the greatest number of people;
• provide equitable access to basic health services;
• extend services to the poor;
• ration expensive and technologies that are not cost-effective.

The policy of ECPs has been promoted by the World Bank (1993). The overall goal is to channel resources into interventions with the highest health impact. Designing an ECP involves the following steps:

1 Estimate the burden of disease for a set of diseases, injuries and risk factors.
2 Select interventions that address those conditions that present the highest burden *and* which can be addressed in a cost-effective way.
3 Estimate the costs of delivering care to the target population.
4 Purchase these care packages from existing providers.

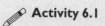 **Activity 6.1**

Table 6.1 provides an analysis of the distribution of the disease burden between children and adults. What does this suggest for the design of an ECP?

Table 6.1 Main cause of disease burden in children and adults in low-income countries in 1990 and cost-effectiveness of the interventions available for their control (Bobadilla et al. 1994)

Disease and injuries	No. of DALYs lost[a] (million)	Main intervention	Cost-effectiveness ($ per DALY)
Children			
Respiratory infections	98 (14.8)[b]	Integrated management of the sick child (IMSC)	30–100
Prenatal morbidity and mortality	95 (14.6)	(a) Prenatal and delivery care	30–100
		(b) Family planning	20–150
Diarrhoeal disease	92 (14.0)	IMSC	30–100
Childhood cluster (diseases preventable through immunization)	65 (10.0)	Expanded programme of immunization EPI-plus[c]	12–30
Congenital melformation	35 (5.4)	Surgical operations	High (unknown)
Malaria	31 (4.7)	IMSC	30–100
Intestinal helminths	17 (2.5)	School health programme	20–34
Protein-energy malnutrition	12 (1.8)	IMSC	30–100
Vitamin A deficiency	12 (1.8)	EPI-plus[c]	12–30
Iodine deficiency	9 (1.4)	Iodine supplementation	19–37
Subtotal	467 (71.0)	–	–
Total DALYs lost	560 (100)	–	–
Adults			
Sexually transmitted diseases (STD) and HIV infection	49.2 (8.9)	Condom subsidy plus IEC[d]	3–18
Tuberculosis	36.6 (6.7)	Short-course chemotherapy	3–7
Cerebrovascular disease	31.7 (5.8)	Case management	High (unknown)
Maternal morbidity and mortality	28.1 (5.1)	Prenatal and delivery care	30–110
Ischaemic heart disease	24.9 (4.5)	Tobacco control programme	35–55
Chronic obstructive pulmonary disease	23.4 (4.3)	Tobacco control programme	35–55
Motor vehicle accidents	18.4 (3.3)	Alcohol control programme	35–55
Depressive disorders	15.7 (2.9)	Case management	500–800
Peri-, endo- and myocarditis and cardiomyopathy	12.4 (2.2)	Case management	High (unknown)
Homicide and violence	12.2 (2.2)	Alcohol control programme	35–55
Subtotal	252.6 (48.6)	–	–
Total DALYs lost	550.0 (100)	–	–

[a] DALYs lost (for specific diseases and the total) are taken from the 1993 World Development Report (r). The total for children and adults include DALYs lost in 1990 due to all diseases and injuries.
[b] Figures in parentheses are percentages.
[c] EPI-plus includes the six vaccines of the Expanded Programme on Immunization (EPI), plus the vaccine against hepatitis B and vitamin A supplementation.
[d] IEC: activities dedicated to information education and communication.

 Feedback

The major part of the burden of disease is concentrated in children and most health problems could be addressed by a small number of highly cost-effective interventions in this area. Intervention in mother and child care is a highly effective way of reducing the burden of disease.

Activity 6.2

According to the model provided in Table 6.2 (opposite):
1   What are the main differences between the ECPs of a low-income and middle-income country? (look at the largest differences in costs per capita)
2   What do the figures suggest about potentially extending the package following economic growth?

Feedback

1 The basic packages are similar except for 'limited care' where there are more complicated conditions and a rider that these conditions may only be treated where 'resources permit'.

2 There is a high demand for services so with economic growth there is scope to extend the ECPs to other cost-effective interventions – such as the management of diabetes, hypertension and some forms of surgery.

Choosing and developing health care provision

In order to set incentives for cost control and quality improvement, defining the terms of the services to be provided (as above) is crucial if purchasing agencies are to avoid the micro-management of providers. Purchasers need to prioritize amongst provider organizations the *unit*, or currency, of care that is being bought – for example, is it an individual intervention or a specified care package; is it for some or all of the population?

A crucial element in how care is provided is size. It is clearly easier for purchasers to make long-term contracts with large providers that look after the greater aspects of care to a population. If the provider unit is small, the purchaser has more difficulty in agreeing on a risk sharing payment mechanism. With smaller units, the purchaser usually must resort to traditional fee-for-service methods of remuneration – but with little ability, therefore, in controlling activity. A wide range of small purchasing units is also costly to administer.

How to purchase services: provider payment methods

The budgeting and provider payment mechanisms are an essential part of the purchaser-provider interaction. You need to be aware that the method of payment establishes different kinds of incentives that providers will react to. There are many methods for paying health care providers, each having a significant impact in terms of the quality and quantity of services provided due to these incentives. There are three main methods (Rice and Smith, 2002):

Table 6.2 Cost-effectiveness of the health interventions (and clusters of interventions) included in the minimum package of health services in low- and middle-income countries (Bobadilla et al. 1994)

Interventions	Cost per beneficiary	Cost per capita	DALYs potentially gained[a] (per 1000 population)	Effectiveness[b]	Cost per DALY($)
Low-income countries					
I *Public health*					
Expanded programme of immunization plus[c]	14.6	0.5	45	0.77	12–17
School health programme	3.6	0.3	4	0.58	20–25
Tobacco and alcohol control programme	0.3	0.3	12	0.14	35–55
AIDS prevention programme[d]	112.2	1.7	35	0.58	3–5
Other public health interventions[e]	2.4	1.4	–	–	–
Subtotal	–	4.2	–	–	14
II *Clinical services*					
Chemotherapy against tuberculosis	500.0	0.6	34	0.51	3–5
Integrated management of the sick child	9.0	1.6	184	0.25	30–50
Family planning	12.0	0.9	7	0.70	20–30
STD treatment	11.0	0.2	26	0.42	1–3
Prenatal and delivery care	90.0	3.8	57	0.42	30–50
Limited care[f]	6.0	0.7	–	0.03	200–300
Subtotal	–	7.8	–	–	–
Total	–	12.0	–	–	–
Middle-income countries					
I *Public health*					
Expanded programme of immunization plus[c]	28.6	0.8	4	0.77	25–30
School health programme	6.5	0.6	5	0.58	38–43
Tobacco and alcohol control programme	0.3	0.3	9	0.14	45–55
AIDS prevention programme[d]	132.3	2.0	15	0.58	13–18
Other public health interventions[e]	5.2	3.1	–	–	–
Subtotal	–	6.9	–	–	–
II *Clinical services*					
Chemotherapy against tuberculosis	275.0	0.2	6	0.51	5–7
Integrated management of the sick child	8.0	1.1	21	0.25	50–100
Family planning	20.0	2.2	6	0.70	100–150
STD treatment	18.0	0.3	3.7	0.42	10–15
Prenatal and delivery care	255.0	8.8	25	0.42	60–110
Limited care[f]	13.0	2.1	–	0.03	400–600
Subtotal	–	14.7	–	–	133
Total	–	21.5	–	–	–

[a] Sum of losses to premature mortality and to disability, including losses to others because of secondary transmission of disease.

[b] Calculated by multiplying efficacy, diagnostic accuracy (when applicable) and compliance.

[c] Plus refers to vaccine against hepatitis B and vitamin A supplementation.

[d] DALYs lost from AIDS include dynamic effects (probability of transmission to others) only in the first year, which understates the value of preventing cases and thus the cost-effectiveness of preventive interventions.

[e] Includes information, communication and education on selected risk factors and health behaviours, plus vector control and disease surveillance.

[f] Includes treatment of infection and minor trauma; for more complicated conditions, includes diagnosis, advice and pain relief, and treatment as resources permit.

1 Full retrospective reimbursement for all expenditure incurred, manifest in *fee for service* (FFS) or item-of-service payment mechanisms.

2 Reimbursement for all activity based on a fixed schedule of fees using a tariff, based on a system of *diagnosis-related groups* (DRGs).

3 Prospective funding based on expected future expenditure using a fixed budget, manifest in salaried employment, devolved budgets and *capitation*.

You might perceive that the three approaches imply a progressive shift of risk from the national funder (fee-for-service) to the provider (devolved and capitated budgets).

Prospective funding based on devolved budgets

In order to contain costs, many health care systems have attempted to move from the former to the latter arrangement. Consequently, a global budget for health care spending is often set, within which care can be purchased. Within the global budget, funders generally devolve a fixed proportion of that budget to providers, but the method of allocation varies:

- It can be undertaken by taking bids from the providers, but such methods encourage providers to overstate needs and raise costs.
- It can be based on political negotiation, though this is open to favouritism and has often proved unsustainable in the long term.
- It can be based on historical precedent and activity, though this does not encourage efficiency and/or innovation.
- It can be based on a more sophisticated measure of local health care needs related to population demographics (capitation). This latter approach is favoured in most high-income countries in Europe, but the problems with developing perceived 'fair shares' through capitation-based formulae has often meant that capitation is mixed with both historic expenditure and some political negotiation.

Given that prospective funding gives a relatively inflexible fixed budget compared to actual expenditure, there is inevitably a process of retrospective variation included in the arrangements. For example, budgets may be renegotiated retrospectively (as in Italy); local taxes may be raised (as in Sweden); co-payments might be levied (as in Finland); or care might be rationed through waiting lists or entitlement changes (implicit in the UK and Norway). You will notice from these strategies that prospective payments tend to under-resource health care against costs.

A *capitation* system puts a monetary value on the 'head' of each member of the population entitled to care. *Risk adjustment* is a key element in the capitation process since capitation funding looks to make an unbiased estimate of expected costs given the characteristics of the population – such as age, sex, income, employment and levels of morbidity. This process is often termed *weighted capitation* to reflect the needs of a specific population. Capitation can be used in both competitive and non-competitive insurance-based funding systems.

Prospective payment

Prospective payment requires a tariff or set of charges to be agreed in advance with providers. The most commonly used method is diagnosis related groups (DRGs). These are a patient classification system that describes the types of patients treated by a hospital (that is, its case mix). DRGs were developed by a group of researchers at Yale University in the late 1960s as a tool to help clinicians and hospitals monitor quality of care and utilization of services. They proved to be so useful that in 1983 they became the system used by Medicare in the USA to pay hospitals.

DRGs categorize patients based on their primary and secondary diagnoses, primary and secondary procedures, age and length of stay. As a way of determining funding, the categories established a uniform cost for each category and funders can then set a maximum amount that would be paid for the care of patients. Under this funding method, hospitals and health care providers are given the incentive to keep health care costs down, since they would experience a profit only if their costs are less than the amount indicated by the DRG category (assuming that their costs were above the DRG rate to begin with). The DRG system of hospital reimbursement is based on prospective payment in which hospitals are compensated for a patient's care based on the qualifying DRG.

Retrospective reimbursement

Retrospective reimbursement is a payment scheme whose level is determined only after services have been provided. It may involve *per diem* payments, a cost/fee per case, and a direct fee for service payment. The main problem with the retrospective reimbursement model of funding is the inability to control provider costs effectively due to weak forms of audit of provider activity. In the USA, for example, the cost of Medicare and Medicaid services (tax-based funding for the old and poor) that began in the 1960s could not be maintained beyond 1983 because federal government income did not provide enough revenue to cover costs. As a consequence a DRG-based funding system was introduced. The 1965–1983 period was recognized as the 'blank check' era since providers received any payment from the federal or state government for patient treatment as long as the requests were 'customary, usual, and reasonable'. As the number of Medicare patients rapidly climbed, the US government could not continue retrospective reimbursement for fear of bankruptcy. A similar policy shift from retrospective reimbursement to prospective payment due to cost inflation occurred in Germany in the 1990s.

Provider payment methods and achieving system objectives

✎ Activity 6.3

Examine the pros and cons of the provider payment mechanisms you have just read about. Which of these approaches do you think can achieve best the following four objectives of a strategic purchaser of health services?

1   to prevent health problems
2   to deliver services
3   to be responsive to people's expectations
4   to contain costs

Complete Table 6.3 to show your understanding of the potential effects on provider behaviour of each mechanism listed.

Table 6.3 Assessing provider behaviour by type of payment mechanism

Provider behaviour / Mechanism	Prevent health problems	Deliver services	Responsive to expectations	Contain costs
Salaried/Global budget				
Capitation				
Diagnostic related payment				
Devolved budget				
Fee-for-service				

Use the following codes to assess each relationship in the table:
+++   very positive effect
++   some positive effect
+/−   little effect
− −   some negative effect
− − −   very negative effect
Source: Adapted from World Health Organization (2000).

Feedback

As Table 6.4 shows, none of the four budgeting mechanisms can achieve all four objectives simultaneously.

Table 6.4 Provider payment mechanisms and provider behaviour

Provider behaviour / Mechanism	Prevent health problems	Deliver services	Responsive to expectations	Contain costs
Salaried/Global budget	++	− −	+/−	+++
Capitation	+++	− −	++	+++
Diagnostic related payment	+/−	++	++	+/−
Devolved budget	++	− −	+/−	+++
Fee-for-service	+/−	+++	+++	− − −

Key:
+++ very positive effect; ++ some positive effect; +/− little effect; − − some negative effect; − − − very negative effect
Source: Adapted from World Health Organization (2000).

It shows that:

- Fee-for-service and prospective payment mechanisms provide strong incentives to deliver services and be responsive to people's demands, but are weaker in containing costs and often do not help the development of preventive care. The French health care system is a classic example of this and reflects their long held policy-level belief in 'la medicine liberale' allowing access to care through social insurance to a wide range of independent practitioners and hospitals. Interestingly, the cost of the system has led the French to reconsider its strategic priorities and to plan a move towards both tax-based funding and capitated payments as ways of controlling costs.
- Capitation mechanisms, salaried service and devolved (global) budgets are more likely to contain costs and invest in preventive care, but are generally less good at responding to patient expectations whilst care deliver is often not able to meet demand, resulting in waiting lists. The English NHS, historically highly cost-efficient in service delivery terms, was a classic example of capitation. However, due to perceived problems in unresponsive services, high waiting lists and problematic access to care, recent reforms have encouraged provider plurality and a 'payments by results' (fee-for-service) system of payment.

Purchasers need to use a combination of payment mechanisms if they are to achieve all their objectives. Free choice of provider by consumers increases responsiveness under all payment systems but particularly under those needing to attract patients to ensure payment from a purchaser (fee-for-service and prospective payment). The French and English diversions away from their historical positions shows how countries have attempted to change provider behaviour to meet a perceived system need – choice and responsiveness, in the case of England, and cost containment, in the case of France.

Internal incentives in funding agencies

If the previous analysis of the potential impact of funding methods has sensitized you to the possible outcomes that can result from different payment methods, you should also be aware that performance of health funding agencies themselves can be influenced by their own internal incentives. The performance of the health funding agencies is dependent on (WHO, 2000):

- The *level of autonomy* that the funding agency has over its overseeing authority or government – for example, over the ability to set contribution levels, design and negotiate contracts and provider pay mechanisms, and to determine purchasing strategies.
- The degree of *accountability* in being responsible for making decisions.
- The degree of *market exposure* in the way revenues are collected (for example, between competing insurers or by a budget allocation). Important for performance is whether governments provide budget supplements for deficits that originate from poor performance.
- The degree of *financial responsibility* for losses, or rights to profits.
- The degree of *unfunded mandates* – the proportion of allocated revenues for which the funding organization is legally responsible but cannot charge fees. For example, to look after the poor or elderly who do not contribute funds to the funding pool.

✏ **Activity 6.4**

In Chapter 5 you were introduced to a range of revenue collection systems. Consider the following four systems:

- administered by a health ministry following general taxation;
- social health insurance administered by a number of government sanctioned insurance agents;
- community insurance administered by a local community from out-of-pocket contributions; and
- a private health insurance company.

To what degree does each system have 'high', 'limited' or 'low' exposure to the forms of internal incentives described above? Complete Table 6.5.

Table 6.5 Assessing exposure of different funding agencies to internal incentives

Organizational form — Internal incentive	Ministry of Health, Finance Department	Social insurance agency	Community pooling organization	Private health insurance
Autonomy (decision-rights)				
Accountability				
Market exposure				
Financial responsibility				
Unfunded mandates				

For each of the incentives (except accountability) make a judgement on whether you think the level of exposure is 'high', 'limited' or 'low'. You can make other judgements if you wish. For the line marked 'accountability', you need to name the accountable authority.

Source: Adapted from World Health Organization (2000).

↻ **Feedback**

All prepaid health financing systems are composed of combinations of the four organizational forms. Each has a different level of exposure to internal incentives. For example, private and community health insurance schemes have more autonomy but are highly exposed to market pressures, carry direct financial risks, and are directly accountable to consumers. Governments and social insurance schemes carry little market exposure and the latter are usually accountable to government. However, the flexibility of their decision-making is low and they carry a high number of unfunded mandates. Your table should look similar to the answers in Table 6.6.

Table 6.6 Exposure of different funding agencies to internal incentives

Internal incentive \ Organizational form	Ministry of Health, Finance Department	Social insurance agency	Community pooling organization	Private health insurance
Autonomy (decision-rights)	Limited	Usually high	High	High
Accountability	Government	Government	Owner/ consumers	Owner/ consumers
Market exposure	None	High if there is competition	High	High
Financial responsibility	None/Low	Low	High	High
Unfunded mandates	High	Low	None/ very low	None/ very low

Source: Adapted from World Health Organization (2000).

External incentives on funding agencies

External incentives are required to govern the way the different types of funding agencies operate. There are three principal external incentive forces:

- *Governance* – the rules and customs that shape the relationship between funding agencies and their owners. Ownership usually provides the right to make ultimate decisions over strategic purchasing plans and to specify and/or limit the services to be purchased.
- *Public policy objectives* – can influence the behaviour of purchasing agencies by providing eligibility criteria for any subsidies (for example, to community or private health insurers) and/or give directives on the way care should be provided (for example, to tackle waiting lists or address a key disease area).
- *Control mechanisms* shape the relationship between the funding agency and the public authorities. For example, through the use of regulation or financial incentives to private insurers, or through the use of top-down hierarchical regulation in the case of nationally administered funds.

Table 6.7 provides a summary of the exposure of the different organizational forms discussed in Activity 6.3 to these external incentives. Evidence from health financing reforms in Latin American countries (Baeza, 1999) shows the potential negative impact of not strengthening control mechanisms (regulation) and shifting to different external incentive instruments when private competitive health insurance is introduced. Cream-skimming (insuring healthier people only) became commonplace, leaving the high cost cases in the public pools and worsening the financial situation of public provision.

Table 6.7 Exposure of different funding agencies to external incentives

Organizational form / External incentive	Ministry of Health, Finance Department	Social insurance agency	Community pooling organization	Private health insurance
Governance	Public, low level of decision rights	Public, variable level of decision rights	Private, high level of decision rights	Private, high level of decision rights
Policy objectives	High	Variable, government and market	None, except when looking for public subsidies	None, except when looking for public subsidies
Control mechanisms	Hierarchical	Mix of hierarchy, regulation and financial incentives	Regulation and some financial incentives	Regulation and some financial incentives

Source: Adapted from World Health Organization (2000).

Summary

Purchasing needs to be effectively managed since the process of making investment priorities effects both the equity and efficiency in the provision of health services. The performance of the system will fall short of its potential if resources are not allocated and spent wisely to gain the best mix of responses to improve health and satisfy needs.

References

Bobadilla, J., Cowley, P., Musgrove, P. and Saxenian, H. (1994) Design, content and financing of an essential national package of health services, *Bulletin of the World Health Organization*, 72(4): 653–62.

Bobadilla, J. and Cowley, P. (1995) Designing and implementing packages of care of essential health services, *Journal of International Development*, 7(3): 543–54.

Rice, N. and Smith, P. (2002) Strategic resource allocation and funding decisions, in E. Mossialos, A. Dixon, J. Figueras, J. Kutzin (2002) *Funding Health Care: Options for Europe*. Buckingham: Open University Press, pp. 250–71.

World Bank (1993) *World Development Report 1993: Investing in Health*, World Bank, Washington.

World Health Organization (2000) *The World Health Report 2000. Health Systems: Improving Performance*, WHO, Geneva.

Further reading

Hutchison, B., Hurley, J., Reid, R. et al. (1999) *Capitation Formulae for Integrated Health Systems: A Policy Synthesis*. Centre for Health Economics and Policy Analysis, McMaster University, Hamilton.

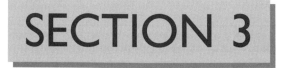

SECTION 3

Managing people

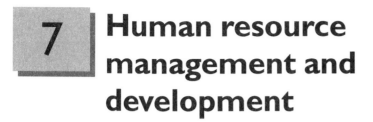

Human resource management and development

Overview

This chapter provides an introduction to the principal activities and tools of human resource management (HRM). In the first part of the chapter, you will examine a model of HRM. You will then examine the opportunities and difficulties of transferring the model to public sector organizations and to low- or middle-income countries. Finally, you will examine the limitations of the human resource development (HRD) model in the health sector and explore ways of improving outcomes by integrating HRM activities.

Learning objectives

After working through this chapter you will be able to:

- identify and assess the principal activities of HRM and the criticisms made of it;
- describe the possible links between HRM and the strategic management of an organization;
- assess to what extent the HRM model is applicable to private and public agencies;
- describe the logical ways in which HRM activities should be integrated;
- outline the benefits of using a systematic approach to HRD in the health sector.

Key terms

Career development The development of a staff member's career within the organization.

Convergence/divergence Processes promoting similarities/differences between countries, or between private and public sector organizations.

Employment relations Management of the relationship between the organization and its staff as a whole.

Human resource development Activities that aim to improve the capacity and quality of the workforce, employee relations, equal opportunities and staff motivation.

Human resource strategy The overall plan for the treatment of staff in an organization.

Job analysis The process of determining the content of jobs and the kinds of skills needed for performing them.

Performance management A systematic approach to the management of individual performance, seeing it in the context of the overall strategy of the organization.

Recruitment and selection The process of finding suitable staff to carry out the jobs identified as necessary for an organization.

What are the activities of human resource management?

As in other areas of public policy and management, human resource management is a contested field of study, with much controversy and many competing models. Reassuringly, however, there is less controversy about the *content* of human resource management. Virtually all writers assume that there is a set of core activities and a body of good practice associated with each of them. The following is a short overview of the topics and concepts which will then be discussed in more detail.

Human resource planning

Human resource planning refers to the group of techniques which enables a manager to plan the staffing of an organization. Organizations, especially large ones, need to forecast their staffing needs. If, for instance, a government has made a commitment to providing universal access to health care, it must estimate how many health care workers to recruit in the different professions in order to realize that commitment. To do so, it will need information on how many professionals are being trained each year and how many leave each year as a result of retirement, death, resignation or for other reasons. Using that information, the Ministry of Health can then forecast its recruitment needs some distance into the future.

Human resource planning often begins with working out the human resource implications of a new health care programme. But even where policies are stable, there may be a need for ongoing estimates of staffing needs as circumstances change. For example, there may be an increase in the number of staff resigning voluntarily, possibly because public sector salaries have fallen behind private sector salaries (as happened in Singapore in the early 1980s). The organization needs to gather data on the scale of the increase so that an appropriate response can be made.

Job analysis

Job analysis refers to the group of techniques that are used to determine the content of jobs and the knowledge, skills and abilities which post-holders require to carry them out. It is different from human resource planning which is carried out at the level of the organization as a whole (or, in the case of a government, at the level of an individual ministry, public enterprise or other large component of the public sector).

Recruitment and selection

Once job analysis has been undertaken, the agency can proceed to recruit staff to fill the jobs it has identified. At the recruitment stage the agency attracts candidates to apply for its jobs; at the selection stage it selects the best person for the job or jobs from among the candidates it has attracted.

Performance management and appraisal

Once the best person has been identified and has started work, agencies often monitor their performance and help them to develop. Some organizations, including health care organizations, have started to take a systematic approach to the management of individual performance, within the context of the overall strategy of the organization: this has come to be called *performance management*. Many organizations have also found it desirable to institute a formal annual review of performance, conducted jointly by the employee and his or her manager: this is called *performance appraisal*.

Career development

Career development refers to the development of the individual's career within the organization. In the course of their career, staff are likely to carry out many different jobs, especially if they are in a professional, administrative or managerial position. Moving to a different job does not necessarily imply making a job application for the new position. While this is one of the ways in which individuals move jobs within an organization, many employers now believe that they should develop the individual careers of their staff so that the health care organization gets the maximum benefit from their services.

Pay management

Deciding how much and in what way staff should be paid is a major part of human resource management. Pay decisions are often based on data about employees' performance, including data from performance management and appraisal procedures.

Employment relations

Employment relations deals with the management of the relationship between the organization and the staff as a whole. In many countries staff are represented by unions, which have a varying extent of influence on personnel issues. However, employment relations are a concern even if the organization is not 'unionized': managers must still decide how the organization is going to communicate with its staff and the extent to which staff should participate in the management of the organization.

Training and development

Although health care professionals have formal educational qualifications, they develop many of their skills through learning on the job and health care organizations often provide additional learning opportunities. These may be off-the-job training courses or work-based development programmes. In either case they are a recognition that staff need to develop new skills, both for their own satisfaction and to meet the needs of the organization.

Employment reform

The growth in public employment in many countries from the 1950s to the 1980s has come to an end. This has been due to budgetary difficulties and, in the specific context of a World Bank, IMF-sponsored structural adjustment programmes. In some countries, reduction in the size of the public sector has been an aspect of the movement away from communism. This has resulted in a need to reduce the number of jobs in publicly funded health services and sometimes also to retrain serving employees. Although experience of job reduction is relatively recent, some evidence of what might constitute good practice is starting to appear.

Activity 7.1

Equal opportunities is an important issue which will be discussed further in Chapter 9. At this stage, think of a health care organization you are familiar with and give a brief account of the equal opportunity policies that are relevant to the above-mentioned HRM activities.

Feedback

Health care organizations are recognizing that they have a responsibility to ensure that their employment practices are in keeping with their general social objectives in promoting the interests of disadvantaged groups, especially women, members of minority ethnic groups and people with disabilities. In other words, they need to ensure that all employees and prospective employees have an *equal opportunity* to make a contribution to the agency's work. This has led to a concern with eliminating unfair discrimination from areas of employment where it may occur, especially in recruitment and selection but also in pay management, training and development.

Strategic HRM and the human cycle: Devanna's model

What is the theory underlying HRM activities? In the mid-1980s a new model of managing staff emerged from high-income countries. It was first applied as an alternative model of personnel management in large business organizations and spread subsequently to public agencies in low- and middle-income countries. This is the so-called human resource management (HRM) model. Because of its prevalence in professional discussion and because of its potential as a vehicle for making improvements in professional practice, you will spend some time learning about it.

Devanna et al (1984) take the activities of human resource management and argue that the practice of HRM activities should be *strategic*, which means that it should be linked to the organization's strategy as developed through its processes of *strategic management*. Strategic management involves consideration of the following:

1 *Mission and strategy*. An organization needs a reason for being (mission) and a sense of how to display materials, information, and people to carry it out (strategy).
2 *Formal structure*. People and tasks are organized to implement the organization's strategy. The organization's formal structure includes its systems of financial accounting and information dissemination.
3 *Human resource system*. People are recruited and developed to do jobs defined by the organization's formal structure; their performance must be monitored and rewards allocated to maintain productivity.

The basic elements of mission and strategy, formal structure and human resource system are *interrelated*. Hence, for a health care organization to accomplish its mission, it must find the optimal structure that is needed to carry out its objectives and attract and retain staff. Organizations need to *adapt* their structures as they evolve, otherwise they may become increasingly inefficient in applying new strategies within outmoded structures.

The human resource cycle

The central concept of the human resource cycle can be visualized in Devanna's model, as shown in Figure 7.1. It shows the four generic functions that are performed by human resource managers in all organizations – selection, appraisal, rewards and development. Organizational performance is a function of these components: *selecting* the right people for the job; *appraising* their performance; *rewarding* them for good performance; and *developing* their skills to improve performance in the future.

You will notice that the link between individual activities and the organization's overall strategy is its *human resource strategy*. Another way of putting this is to say that organizational strategy is first translated into a human resource strategy, and the latter is then translated into the different human resource activities which are its practical manifestation.

There is a second type of integration implicit in Devanna's model – that of *integration of activities*. While strategic integration refers to links between the HR activities and the organization's strategy, integration of activities refers to links between the HR activities themselves and the fact that the conduct of one HR task may influence the conduct of another. So, for instance, the conduct of selection may influence the conduct of rewards, or vice versa.

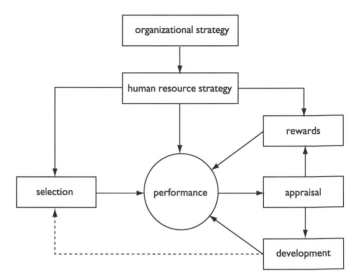

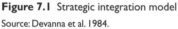

Figure 7.1 Strategic integration model
Source: Devanna et al. 1984.

✏️ **Activity 7.2**

Think of your own organization and try to imagine how a strategic approach to HRM might enable the organization to meet its mission and strategy.

1   What do you think are the features of strategic human resource management?
2   How would taking a strategic HRM approach affect the practice of staff selection? Take, for example, the selection of community health workers for a mother and child health programme in a country with high infant mortality.

↻ **Feedback**

1 Human resource management should be brought in line with the overall strategic management of the organization. In the first instance, the organization should articulate a human resource philosophy. This might indicate the extent to which the organization prefers to promote from within rather than recruit from outside, or it might indicate the extent to which the organization prefers to emphasize the individual or the group as the unit of production. In the second instance, it means ensuring that the individual human resource components are also aligned with the organization's overall strategy.

2 You might have identified three strategic concerns:

• designing a selection system that matches the organization's strategy;
• monitoring the internal flow of personnel to match emerging business strategies;
• matching key executives to business strategies.

For example, the strategic goal of organizing a successful mother and child health programme creates a need to select female health care workers who are respected by the local community and who can effectively communicate health issues to women in their environment.

The outcomes of strategic HRM: understanding Guest's model

The strategic HRM model you have just considered has been extended. David Guest (1989), for example, outlines an extended version by listing the distinctive outcomes associated with it. These include:

1 *Strategic integration*. HRM policies and practices are fully coherent, accepted and used by line managers.
2 *Commitment*. The goal of binding employees to the organization through commitment to high performance.
3 *Flexibility*. The organization is adaptive and receptive to innovation and change through job enrichment and workforce multi-skilling.
4 *Quality*. Staff of high quality, both employees and managers, are recruited.

Guest's theory has features in common with Devanna's model: the HR activities (Guest calls them 'policies') and the notion of strategic integration. Thus, to achieve HRM outcomes, best practice in conventional HR activities listed on the left of Table 7.1 needs to be achieved.

Table 7.1 Theory of human resource management (Guest 1989)

HRM policies	Human resource outcomes	Organizational outcomes
Organization/job design		*High*
	Strategic integration	Job performance
Management of change		
		High
Recruitment and selection	Commitment	Problem-solving
		Change and innovation
Appraisal, training and development	Flexibility/adaptability	*High*
		Cost-effectiveness
Reward systems	Quality	
		Low
		Turnover
		Absence and grievances
Leadership/Culture/Strategy		

There are also additional elements to Guest's model, including the role of a *strong organizational culture*, *key leadership* and a *conscious strategy*, which combined provide the cement to full and effective utilization of human resources. A particularly important part of the model is that HR should be managed by line managers and not personnel managers. This suggests that while there may be specialist aspects of human resource management best left to specialist staff, the management of staff needs to be an integral part of any manager's job.

In achieving HRM outcomes (on the right-hand side of Table 7.1), a set of conditions must be in place for the model to be implemented successfully. This is needed, especially in health care organizations, to overcome the individualist nature of professionals working within them and the need to engender commitment and strategic integration. The five conditions (or constraints to overcome) are:

1 *Corporate leadership.* A willingness at the top of an organization to support the values through which HRM strategies will succeed.
2 *Strategic vision.* A shared view across the organization between managers and staff that HRM is a key part of the corporate strategy.
3 *Technological/production feasibility.* HRM is difficult where large numbers of staff are employed in short-cycle, repetitive production line tasks. For HRM to be effective, such constraining structures need to become more flexible and adaptive.
4 *Employee/industrial relations feasibility.* Established worker and managerial attitudes, often enshrined in union activity, can be a major barrier to the persuit of HRM yet need to be addressed to foster flexibility and commitment.
5 *Ability to get HRM policies in place.* Personnel departments often have a poor record in translating HRM strategies into operational processes.

Activity 7.3

What is the importance of staff commitment and line management ownership? Illustrate your answer with an example from health services.

Feedback

It is desirable that managers should be involved in the selection of staff to do the jobs for which they will be accountable. This is partly because the line manager is in a better position than some distant human resource specialist to know what the job requires and partly because the manager's involvement increases his or her commitment to making the appointment a success.

Many health services are highly centralized and line managers have little real influence on new appointments, judgements about performance, pay decisions and assessments of training needs. While types of human resource decisions for which line managers and human resource specialists are responsible will differ with the type of agency (for example, a hospital or an insurance company), the principle of line manager ownership of human resource decisions which affect staff remains valid and important.

As Table 7.1 shows, the skilful practice of individual activities (such as recruitment and selection) leads to human resource outcomes (such as commitment), which in turn contribute to organizational outcomes (such as high job performance and cost-effectiveness). Proponents of the model point to examples of organizations which have used it to improve their performance. The following is an example on how the elements of it were applied by one such organization (British Airways) in its transition from the public to the private sector.

Applying the HRM model at British Airways

The human resource policies followed by British Airways (BA) in the early 1980s, just before and just after its privatization by the British government, are an example of the application of some of the HRM concepts you have learned about. The airline had been unprofitable in public ownership: in the financial year 1981/2, for instance, it suffered a severe financial loss. While some of the measures taken were drastic and short-term – in particular, a reduction in the number of jobs from 60,000 to 38,000 over only a couple of years – others focused on improving staff performance through some of the methods just discussed, including measures aimed at changing the culture of the airline and increasing line manager ownership of human resource issues. You will focus here on its attempts to improve the quality of its service.

In 1982, following market research which showed that the airline's passengers were dissatisfied with its service, BA launched an extensive campaign for all of its 12,000 staff who had direct contact with customers. Up to 150 staff at a time, from baggage-handlers to engineers and pilots, took part in customer service events. The campaign was later extended, so that eventually all of BA's staff attended one of the events. 'Customer First' teams were set up to look at ways of improving customer service. Membership of the teams cut across organizational boundaries, with staff from different sections working together. In 1992, 75 such teams were active.

Further market research shows that customer satisfaction with the quality of BA's service increased. Since BA moved from financial loss to spectacular profit over the period when these initiatives took place (in February 1995 it reported record profits of £443 million, with passengers totalling 23.7 million), its financial success was partly attributed to its human resource initiatives. However, it should be noted that some problems remained. Despite its HR initiatives, a staff survey in 1992 showed that staff rated BA poorly as an employer for sustaining a working environment that attracts, retains and develops committed employees, suggesting that commitment, one of the elements in Guest's model, remains a problem. In mid-1997, BA also lost a damaging strike following an attempt to impose a new pay deal on its staff without negotiation.

Applying the HRM model

The experience of British Airways is positive evidence of the pay-off that comes from applying the HRM model appropriately. It is only recently, however, that worthwhile attempts have been made to study the effects of the HRM model in practice and they have not necessarily been positive or conclusive. This is for several reasons, including:

1 *The ideological character of the HRM model.* It has been alleged that a major function of the HRM model is to bolster the power of managers over workers, and the model is closely related to changes in some OECD countries in the 1980s, notably the UK and the USA, where the election of right-wing governments led to changes in legislation and in the climate of management in organizations, which increased managers' control (Guest, 1989). However, this argument is inconclusive. Recent research in Britain shows that companies using HRM practices tend also to be companies where staff are represented by

trade unions – hardly an indication that the HRM model bolsters the power of managers over workers.

2   *The un-strategic nature of management.* It has been argued that decisions are often short-term and frequently finance-led, with human resource considerations appearing only as a second-order consideration. Such decisions militate against the strategic integration which is the central feature of the HRM model.

3   *The low take-up of the HRM model.* Lastly, and perhaps following from the above points, the new HRM model has been adopted in its entirety only in a minority of even private sector firms in OECD countries.

Public and private sector applications of the HRM model

The evidence for the application of the HRM model in the private sector in high-income countries is mixed. What prospect is there of its application in the very different conditions of the public sector in low- and middle-income countries? The answer depends largely on the extent of the similarity between organizations in the public and private sectors, and between organizations in high-income and in low- and middle-income countries.

Activity 7.4

Taking the application of HRM as a yardstick, are public and private sector organizations becoming more alike, and are organizations in high-income countries becoming more like those in low- and middle-income countries?

Feedback

Some argue that the changes that have taken place (roughly since the beginning of the 1980s) have reduced the differences that previously existed and that the direction of change is towards further reduction: this is the *convergence view*. At the other extreme are those who argue that important differences persist which show no sign of diminishing: this is the *divergence view*. Convergence and divergence arguments have been developed separately in relation to differences between the private and public sectors, and between OECD and non-OECD countries.

Applying the HRM model in the public sector

In the case of the public sector, the convergence argument is that the introduction of new public management, with its emphasis on general management skills at the expense of professional priorities, has blurred the distinction between private and public sectors (Dunleavy and Hood, 1994). This can be seen in areas like pay management. In late 1998, the government of Ghana was decentralizing the payment of its health care staff, giving greater responsibility for pay decisions to local managers as part of the reorganization of its health services, bringing it into line with the practice of many large private companies. On the other hand, the divergence argument is that the fundamentally different character of the public sector means that the political logic of government will override the agency logic of new public management, and that political control will be reasserted over devolved management units, restoring the distinctiveness of public management (Ferner, 1994).

Applying the HRM model in low- and middle-income countries

In the case of low- and middle-income countries, the convergence argument is that differences between such countries and high-income countries are the product of technological, economic, legal and political conditions, and that because those conditions are converging rapidly, they can be discounted as an influence on organizational behaviour (Negandhi and Prasad, 1987). The divergence argument is that there are deep-seated cultural differences between countries which render Western management theories, such as the HRM model, inapplicable in different cultural settings (Hofstede, 1980).

Case study: HRM in China

Recent political and economic development has brought public-sector organizations in China closer to their Western counterparts. But has HRM been applied in a way that sees employees 'as a valuable resource to be effectively developed and not merely as a cost of production'? (Warner, 1995). As Table 7.2 shows, in the past in

Table 7.2 Changes in HRM practices in China

Activity	Past practice	Present practice
Human resource planning	little planning at the level of small enterprise; planning at provincial and municipal levels; (mis-) allocation of graduates at national level	past practice still applies; greater autonomy in joint ventures and foreign-owned firms
Recruitment and selection	selection decisions made at a level above the plant; promotion based on seniority	joint ventures have more freedom
Performance management and appraisal	emphasis on group norms of production	(unspecified) improvement in practice
Pay management	ideology emphasized rather than rewards in past; rewards were egalitarian	growing emphasis on material rewards; bonuses paid to productive plants, not to individuals
Employment relations	Socialist-type enterprise-based unions; worker participation widespread	changing role for unions; no unions in foreign-owned firms
Training and development	training previously narrow	compulsory training for managers being introduced
Employment reform	dismissals rare; lifetime employment usual	some use of fixed-term contracts; flexible working in joint ventures

Source: M. Warner (1995)

China there was no human resource planning at the level of individual enterprises and graduates were allocated by a central ministry rather than selected. However, we should be careful not to assume that difference inevitably acts as a limitation on applying good practice that comes from somewhere else. For example, centralization of management decision-making, a characteristic of many Chinese organizations, is conducive to taking a strategic view of human resources. Similarly, worker participation and the identification of workers with their workplaces conform to some recent thinking on employment relations, which emphasizes the importance of participation and commitment.

There is evidence that changes in Chinese government policies have had an impact on the current practice of human resource management. To take two examples, individual enterprises now have more freedom to recruit the staff they want and there is more training for managers. The convergence argument seems to be supported, therefore, by the introduction of approaches such as flexible working which are practised elsewhere.

However, there is also contrary evidence, at least in relation to one of the major areas of human resource management – that of pay management. A research study by Easterby-Smith and Yuan (1995) compared human resource management in China and the UK and found that whilst the ratio between the top and bottom earners in four UK companies varied from 20:1 to 40:1; in China it was never higher than 4:1. The researchers attributed the difference to the high level of individualism in the UK and the need to maintain harmonious relations within organizations in China in line with cultural norms.

Activity 7.5

Think about the application of the HRM model to the public sector in your country.

To what extent are the conditions conducive to implementation of the HRM model? Have there been recent changes in the role of unions, in reward schemes, or in the relationship between central and decentralized organization?

Feedback

Your answer will differ with your country and experience. Many public sector organizations have undergone changes in HRM practice, often without applying a coherent model. To a varying extent, HRM responsibilities have been transferred to line managers. Privatization of large public sector agencies was influential in introducing a new approach to HRM. Many societies have experienced changes in industrial relations, often with a weakened role of unions.

The HRM model in practice

While the implementation of a comprehensive HRM model may be problematic, there still remains a body of good practice in each of its activities. The notion of good practice has some problems of its own, and your critical skills will be needed to appraise it. Good practice can be implemented even where a strategic HRM approach is not possible. For example, a health care organization may not be able to develop all the potential links between different human resource activities but may still be in a position to use some of them in a piecemeal way.

For practical purposes you should keep in mind:

- there is a body of good practice in each of the HRM activities which you are going to study (the principle of good practice);
- HRM can be arranged to form a logical sequence (the principle of logical sequence);
- HRM is strengthened by linking activities together (the principle of integration of activities).

✎ Activity 7.6

Suppose you have to organize a new health care programme. Draw a flow diagram of the logical sequence of the HRM activities (refer to the list of activities presented earlier) during planning and implementation of the service.

↻ Feedback

Your diagram should look similar to Figure 7.2. The sequence begins with *human resource planning*, logically the first activity the organization carries out when it wishes to identify its overall staffing needs. Having done that, you move from the level of overall needs to the level of the individual job and use *job analysis* to identify the content of those jobs. You are now in a position to undertake *recruitment and selection* and to identify suitable candidates to fill the jobs. Once the successful candidates are in post, you need to monitor their performance and give them the opportunity to develop, which you can do through formal activities of *performance management and appraisal*, as well as through day-to-day work and interaction between employees and managers. The outcome of the annual appraisal interview may affect the individual's pay: if the outcome is positive, pay may increase. Thus appraisal may lead into decisions about *pay management*. It may also lead to decisions about *training and development* since training needs can be identified through appraisal. Through the process of *employment reform*, the health programme may realize that it no longer needs, or can afford, some of its jobs. At any stage in the sequence, the organization that is responsible for the health care programme may need to communicate its policies to its staff, or respond to their concerns: this is the domain of *employment relations*.

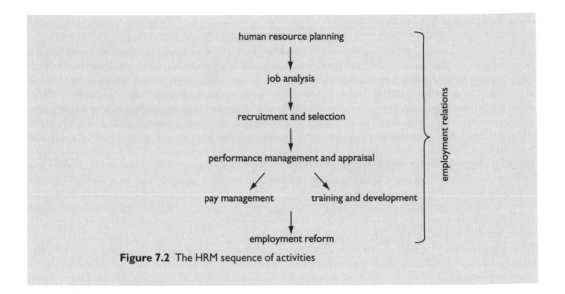

Figure 7.2 The HRM sequence of activities

It is important to keep in mind that the sequence is logical, not chronological. In real life, many of these activities go on simultaneously and there is some arbitrariness. Pay management, for instance, could equally be placed between job analysis and recruitment and selection. Training needs may arise earlier in the process of programme implementation. Employment relations cannot be fitted into the sequence: there may be interaction between representatives of the employer and the employee on any of the other activities (though in practice the greatest interaction is usually on pay).

Integration of HRM activities

Integration of HRM activities refers to how the conduct of one HR task may influence the conduct of another, so that the contribution that individual activities make to the organization is strengthened by linking them together. So, for instance, the contribution of recruitment and selection may be strengthened by developing its links with performance management. Thus, job analysis data gathered as part of a pay determination exercise should also be used when the agency is recruiting staff to those jobs. It should also be made available to the staff themselves and to the managers of those staff, for whom it is a valuable tool in managing staff performance. Of course, in a large public sector where the Ministry of Finance is responsible for pay decisions and the Ministry of Health is responsible for recruitment and selection of staff, this is hard to do; but the point remains valid. Table 7.3 shows potential integrative links between HRM activities, but it does not show a link between recruitment and selection, and employment reform.

Table 7.3 Integrating human resource activities

HRP	JA	R & S	PM	Pay	T & D	E Ref	E Rel
Human resource planning	HRP basis for JA at organization level				HRP may highlight training need	HRP as approach to employment reform	HR plans may be discussed with union
Job analysis		JA is basis of selection decisions	JA gives agenda for appraisal interview	gradings are based on JA	JA used to identify training needs	JA used to identify redundant jobs	may be disputes over job boundaries
Recruitment and selection			information gained in selection feeds into appraisal	pay may be discussed in the interview	selection may identify training needs		may be disputes over selection
Performance management				pay may be based on appraisal	training needs identified through PA	appraisal ratings used to retrench	disputes possible over appraisal
Pay management					training may increase pay	close link between reform of pay and employment	pay negotiated with unions
Training and development						retraining an element of employment reform	disputes over training entitlement
Employment reform							employment reform discussed with union
Employment relations							

HRM in the health sector

You saw earlier that there are elements of both convergence and divergence in the development of human resource management in the private sector of high-income countries and the public sector in low- and middle-income countries. How, then, does the HRM model work in the health sector, which is one of the largest public agencies in many countries? And how can its activities be applied to the heterogeneous structure of the health sector with a mix of private and public organizations?

Transferring HRM methods to health systems is problematic since all the methods (or tools) that you will come across have been developed in particular contexts or to serve particular purposes and may need to be adapted before they can be used in health care. You need to be critically aware of possible limitations imposed by the circumstances in which they were first developed and be willing to adapt them when necessary. Moreover, critical adaptation may on occasion mean rejection. There are many situations where a standard HRM technique is the right one to use in health care organizations. But there are others where it is not, or where no technique exists because the problem that you confront is not recognized in the professional literature.

Case study: adapting HRM techniques in Bangladesh

In 1998, Bangladesh adopted, in its Fifth Health and Population Programme, a sector-wide approach to HRM to ensure an adequate supply of health and family planning staff, to strengthen education and training of health workers, and to support a better performance management and personnel administration. A 'needs-orientated approach to HRD' is seen as an essential part of a strategy to improve health service delivery and equity of access to care. Although critics may say that this is not very different from good practice in personnel management, the example demonstrates (apart from the government rhetoric) that the idea of a strategic approach to HRM is filtering into national health policies.

Human resource development in health care

The most important human resource issues in the health sector are very similar to those discussed earlier in this chapter. These include the ability to reduce costs by improving staff skill-mix; improving staff performance through mechanisms for rewards and sanctions; and improving equity in the distribution of services by providing appropriate incentives to control staff supply. Health care organizations must invest in the development of HR policy and planning capacity to achieve their goals.

Ultimately, the rationale for using HRM models is to improve health outcomes by improving efficiency. In health sector reforms, strategies rely on the development of human resources since the efficiency of the workforce depends largely on the way it is managed. Human resource development (HRD) is the process that is concerned with the different functions involved (planning, managing, supporting performance) and the key overall aim is to get the right people with the right skills and motivation in the right place at the right time.

Summary

In this chapter you have gained an overview of the core activities of HRM and you have seen that, in the new HRM model of staff management, human resource activities are linked to human resource outcomes (strategic integration, commitment, flexibility/adaptability, quality, line manager ownership and culture), which in turn are linked to organizational outcomes (such as high job performance). You have studied the application of the HRM model and examined the principles of logical sequencing and integration of HRM activities. Finally, you were introduced to the application of HRD in the health sector. In the following four chapters you will embark on the study of the individual activities that are the major components of human resource management, starting in Chapter 8 with human resource planning and forecasting.

References

Devanna, M., Fombrun, C. and Tichy, N. (1984) A framework for strategic human resource management, in C. Fombrun, N. Tichy and M. Devanna (eds) *Strategic Human Resource Management*. New York: John Wiley, pp. 33–51.

Dunleavy, P. and Hood, C. (1994) From old public administration to new public management, *Public Money and Management*, 14(3): 34–43.

Easterby-Smith, M. and Yuan, P. (1995) How culture sensitive is HRM? A comparative analysis of practice in Chinese and UK companies, *International Journal of Human Resource Management*, 6: 115–9.

Ferner, A. (1994) The state as employer, in R. Hyman and A. Ferner (eds) *New Frontiers in European Industrial Relations*, pp. 52–79. Oxford: Blackwell.

Guest, D. (1989) Personnel and HRM: can you tell the difference?, *Personnel Management*, January: 48–51.

Hofstede, G. (1980) Motivation, leadership and organisation: do American theories apply abroad?, *Organizational Dynamics*, 9: 42–63.

Negandhi, A. and Prasad, S. B. (1987) Convergence in organisational practices: an empirical study of industrial enterprises in developing countries, in C. Lammers (ed.) *Legal Principles*. New York: John Wiley.

Warner, M. (1995) Human Resource Management 'with Chinese Characteristics', *The International Journal of Human Resource Management*, 4(1): 13–8.

8 Human resource planning: forecasting demand and supply

Overview

This chapter introduces you to human resource planning (HRP) in health care services, both at the organizational and the sector level. You will first look at precedence, analogy and professional judgement as pragmatic approaches to HRP and then at a conceptual framework for a strategic approach to HRP. You will then consider how to achieve appropriate staffing levels based on practical examples of demand and supply forecasting, including how a human resources plan is prepared.

Learning objectives

After working through this chapter you will be able to:

- describe how HRP can contribute to strategic results;
- assess the information required to support HRP;
- outline a framework for HRP;
- define demand and supply forecasting, and how to structure such forecasts;
- assess the strengths and weakness of a top-down versus bottom-up approach to budgeting staff expenditure;
- calculate staff turnover and stability rates.

Key terms

Analogy Making decisions about staffing by considering the structure of another health care organization.

Managerial judgement Decision-making on the basis of specific criteria developed for the purpose when precedent and analogy are not helpful; ideally a needs-based approach that takes into account historically developed structures and stakeholders' interests.

Performance indicators Financial and non-financial measures used for monitoring activity levels, efficiency and quality of service provision by comparing actual with expected results.

Precedent An approach to decision-making about staffing needs based on previous custom and practice.

Stability rate A measure of how well a staff category is standing up to erosion in its numbers due to wastage from the organization.

> **Staff turnover** Staff wastage, or changes in staff levels over time; they can be due either to avoidable circumstances (such as dissatisfaction with poor management) or to unavoidable events (such as retirement, illness).

Introduction

HRP is driven by a concern that the work achieved in jobs should contribute to the strategic goals of the particular organization, both now and in the future. It also addresses how jobs may be filled by appropriately qualified people at the right time so that this aim can be achieved. Given that managers are primarily responsible for these two tasks, HRP supports managerial decision-making to make effective the acquisition, deployment, utilization, development and retention of people at work, by addressing such issues as:

- How many staff are required in the organization?
- What are the staffing implications of a new decentralization policy?
- Should there be concerns about the rate of staff wastage?
- Is it time to start a graduate recruitment programme?
- What can be done to promote more women into senior positions?
- How many staff need to be trained to introduce a new technology or programme?

HRP is applicable to all types of organizations within the health sector – publicly funded organizations, ministries, insurance agencies, NGOs (non-governmental organizations), and private companies. It is distinct from national or sectoral human resource planning because it is applied in a management context, although some of the forecasting methods may be similar.

Demand forecasting

HRP starts by considering staffing levels in relation to strategic goals and the volumes of work they imply. This aspect of planning is known as *demand forecasting* (that is, establishing the number of posts required) and you will note that it is critically related to financial questions about the affordability of the workforce. Demand forecasting is important because training and developing the workforce is expensive.

The methods used to control the supply of doctors vary greatly between health systems. Most countries have abandoned the *laissez-faire* approach to medical supply and try to exert some kind of control in planning the numbers of doctors. Basically, there are two different approaches: restricting access to medical education and restricting access to medical practice.

In the UK and Sweden, where the state is virtually a monopoly employer of doctors (either through direct employment or via exclusive contracts), the number of places in medical schools and the posts in health services have been planned for decades. Other countries, such as Italy or Germany, have greater difficulty in restricting access to medical school, because exercising control of medical education would infringe the guaranteed right to higher education which is part of the constitution. These countries regulate access to practice, with the consequence that medical unemployment is relatively high.

Wastage of trained health care professionals is not uncommon in countries which produce more professionals than can be absorbed by the local labour market. In this situation many professionals migrate to find work abroad. Some countries rely on immigrant health workers to mitigate shortages in staff supply. Oversupply is tolerated as the remittances of health care workers who have emigrated provide support to the national economy.

Activity 8.1

Deciding staffing levels and then recruiting, deploying and developing staff to meet new organizational demands has long been a part of managers' tasks. Thinking in pragmatic terms, what approaches to deciding on staffing levels would you consider taking in staffing a new health centre?

Feedback

Normally, you have three options to choose from, as follows.

1 *Precedent.* 'When we last opened a health centre, how did we staff it?' Large, well-established organizations may or may not have formal human resource plans, but they almost certainly have *custom and practice* – that is, they have evolved staffing policies incrementally, whether or not those policies are written down. Precedent oils the wheels of classic bureaucracies and determines expectations of what may (or should) happen in the future. If you staff your new health centre without reference to precedents, you may create a salary anomaly, which staff in other parts of the organization may not find acceptable.

2 *Analogy.* Where precedents do not exist, managers often fall back on analogies. Thus, when you have never had this type of centre before and are establishing this one as a first step towards decentralizing, then no precedent exists. You might plan staffing by analogy with the structure of another health care organization, and relate the staffing establishment to that. This may feel fair – that is the interested parties are satisfied that the staffing outcome is equitable.

3 *Individual managerial judgement.* Even the largest, most stable and well-established organizations have to make a leap in the dark from time to time. Precedent and analogy may give way to a new rationale based on managerial judgement. Even without a full planning diagnosis, the health centre may be staffed according to specific criteria developed for the purpose. Ideally, you would take a needs-based approach, informed by demographic and epidemiological data which take into account historically grown structures and stakeholders' interests.

The usefulness of human resource planning in organizations

Managers at organizational level are rarely involved in planning sector-wide human resources. In the general management literature, for example, there is a long-standing interest in managerial judgement going back to the work of Vickers (1965). The judgement of an effective manager is based on his or her accumulated experience and tacit intelligence, expressed in problem-solving skills which have developed over years.

However, managerial judgement may be insufficient in the more complex context of a changing environment or in conditions of financial constraint, because it does not generate a diagnosis of sufficient depth to allow different options to be considered. HRP ensures that priorities are analysed adequately and options made available to managers. It seeks to be flexible in relation to changing needs and is increasingly focused on staff groups with skills in high demand. Planning methods, therefore, have moved towards supporting managers' decisions through a diagnostic approach that generates information and possible strategic options.

Establishing a strategic framework for human resource planning

A strategic framework for HRP is shown in Figure 8.1. This establishes the links between strategic objectives and numbers of posts required (demand) and indicates strategic options to ensure that projected vacancies are filled by appropriately qualified people (supply). Data needs, analytical inputs and decisions in HRP are implied by the connections between the boxes of the chart. The diagram shows five stages for human resource planning.

Each stage of the HRP process can be described as follows:

Investigating Boxes 1–5: building up awareness of the personnel situation, in particular identifying key problems, opportunities and staff groups which should take precedence in planning work.

Forecasting Boxes 6–8: making predictions; in particular, examining possible courses of action based on different sets of assumptions. Work at this stage can indicate further analyses and discussions required at the investigating stage. A draft document with questions and options for discussion by managers is produced at this stage. The key task is to understand how demand (number of posts required to undertake the predicted volume of work) may be reconciled with supply (availability of staff qualified to do the work), and how that can be planned.

Planning Boxes 9 and 10: agreeing on strategies and translating them into targets for priority action. Targets require specified timeframes and a given allocation of resources to implement them, and also criteria for monitoring implementation. Strategies across a range of areas are checked for consistency before commitment to a specific course of action.

Implementing Boxes 11–14: deploying resources to meet targets.

Monitoring and evaluating Box 15: recording and communicating to managers data on progress of implementation.

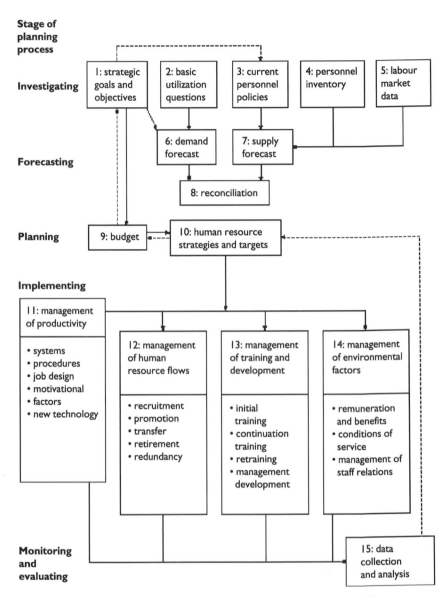

Figure 8.1 A strategic framework for human resource planning (Brahman 1988)

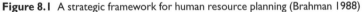

✎ Activity 8.2

What are the information requirements for establishing a human resource plan for a hospital? What data sources might you access?

Feedback

All planning relies on a good supply of information about the hospital and its environment. Information can be used to inform, diagnose problems, assess performance and plan for the future. A potential list of sources includes:

- staff number and whole-time equivalents
- staff grades
- locations
- length of service
- age
- sex
- absenteeism
- staff turnover
- skills and qualifications held
- workloads
- staff costs (basic and additional)
- sources of recruits
- destinations of leavers
- patterns of work

Much of the data will come from the personnel information system of the hospital. Basic personnel data are indispensable for assessing stocks and flows in a demand forecast. To forecast supply, you would need to also access external information sources. You may have informal contacts with education providers and be informed, for example, about the local supply of nursing graduates. Knowledge of the local labour market is essential for assessing recruitment options. Demographic changes and population migration in the catchment area may affect demand for services and thus staffing needs. For example, fewer children in the area may lead to downsizing of the paediatric department.

A simple workforce plan

Managers are often asked to predict the demand for health care professionals in the future. Strike's (1995) simple demand forecasting model (Table 8.1) is one example of assessing the current *stocks* of staff from which to derive a forecast from the balance of intake and losses.

Table 8.1 Demand forecasting table

Year	One	Two	Three	Four	Five
Stock	50	50	48	52	58
Intake	10	10	12	16	20
Losses	10	12	8	10	12
Balance	50	48	52	58	66
Requirements	50	55	60	65	70
Additional demand	–	7	8	7	4

Source: A. Strike (1995)

Suppose that the numbers in Table 8.1 refer to nurses in a community hospital. The terms of Strike's model can then be explained as follows:

Stocks The current number of staff employed is needed to start the plan. The figure in year one is factual, 50 nurses, the other are future estimates.

Intake In previous years demand will have been forecast and the numbers of nurses in training should have reflected that demand. The numbers in the intake row reflect the predicted numbers of qualified nurses that will be designated to the community hospital. In the example, demand is increasing so there is increasing out-turn from the nurse training programme.

Losses Historical turnover rates, together with the age of staff, enables a prediction to be made of the number of nurses likely to leave the hospital in subsequent years.

Balance The balance of nurses is a function of simply adding the intake numbers and subtracting the losses. For predictive purposes, this number forms the basis of the stock of nurses available for the next year.

Requirements Workload and service changes in the community hospital can effect the numbers of nurses required. The model in this case is predicting the need for a steady growth in the need for nurse numbers in the future.

Additional demand The last row is the difference between the balance and the required numbers of nurses. This figure predicts whether there is likely to be an oversupply or, as in this case, a shortage of skilled nurses over the planning period. In such a case, managers may seek to recruit nurses from outside the traditional employment pool (for example, from other regions or even overseas), or delay service expansion plans until the required number of nurses is available.

Forecasting demand to improve performance

Demand forecasting incorporates the principle that it is only worthwhile forecasting a future number of posts in an occupational category when a rationale for current and projected work performances has been developed and accepted. For example, it would make no sense to forecast the need for 20 nurses, when the job could be done as easily by 15. And vice versa, if staff estimates are too low, the forecast would be unrealistic and more staff would be needed for implementation of the organizational plan. Thus, the rationale for demand forecasting rests on a diagnostic approach, with four basic questions addressed to the work situation investigated:

- What factors determine workload?
- How can staff performance be measured?
- How can performance be improved?
- What method should be used to forecast numbers of posts required in future?

Answering these four questions requires discussion amongst the managers and staff immediately involved in the work. Their experience of working practices, the technology used and staff productivity provide a useful guide for understanding current performance and forecasting future staffing needs. The manager's responsibility for performance is important and, for future staffing needs, it is critical. In most circumstances the manager is the most appropriate person to make a demand forecast based on assessing current staff utilization, judging the potential for improvement and forecasting total work volumes.

Activity 8.3

You are asked to prepare a demand forecast for medical assistants in a rural health district. Medical assistants cover a range of activities, such as simple treatments and vaccinations, in a health centre under supervision of a doctor.

1 What factors determine workload?
2 How can staff performance be measured?
3 How can performance be improved?
4 What method should be used to forecast numbers of posts required in future?

Feedback

1

- number of patients registered
- number of beds in the health centre
- size of the population to be covered
- number of supporting staff
- staff costs (basic and additional)

2

- number of patients who attended in the given period (activity)
- number of patients discharged
- time taken to treat a patient
- staff punctuality

3

- improved diagnosis
- more timely treatment
- better staff organization and motivation

4

- number of posts related to the population and epidemiological data

Forecasting using specific indicators of performance

The last of the four essential questions above referred to the forecasting method based on indicators relevant to the type of work involved. The indicator method to establish the future number of posts in a particular job category proceeds through four stages:

Stage 1 Identify an indicator related to the work of the staff category which can be used for forecasting purposes. The indicator should be:

- quantifiable;
- understood by employees, their managers and others concerned, particularly as to how its value is calculated;
- able to be used for negotiation with staff in establishing adequate performance levels if the organizational climate allows this (seeking an agreement on the value to be attached to the indicator);
- based on data easily accessible in the organization's information systems.

For the performance and time indicators only, a current value attached to the indicator provides a means to discuss how well the relevant manager is performing. In this case, the indicator directly links current accountability for performance with future prospects for improvement.

Stage 2 Establish a current value for the indicator which represents the average workload to be expected from each post (or if appropriate from a team).

Stage 3 Determine a value for the indicator which can be used for forecasting purposes, after examining the major factors that may influence how that work is performed in the future.

Stage 4 Relate the future indicator value to the total level of activity expected, to establish the number of posts (teams) required in the category under review, for example:

- number of posts required (performance indicator) = forecast of future *level of activity*
- number of posts required (time indicator) = *total time* demanded by standard *tasks* (in a specified calendar duration) / time offered by one post or team (in same calendar period).

Note that 'time offered by one post or team (in same calendar period)' is the aggregate number of hours available for work (excluding holidays, sickness allowance, training days, set-up periods, and so on).

The indicator method relies very much on those involved in forecasting sharing an agreed feel for the situation. Many sources of information are utilized and shared to identify the average level of performance expected from a jobholder or team, in given technical and environmental circumstances. Much of this information is possibly incomplete at the time of the decision, or estimates are difficult to make, but the decision will be legitimate if those involved consider it acceptable.

Human resource planning and the budget

HRP is only likely to be effective if budgetary guidelines and constraints are incorporated within organizational plans. There are two approaches to determining staffing levels: a bottom-up versus a top-down approach. Each has its strengths and weaknesses.

The bottom-up approach

The bottom-up approach to demand forecasting is aligned to decentralized decision-making. Once organizational goals have been translated into unit objectives, the managers in charge of decentralized units (such as district hospitals or health centres) determine personnel requirements. The strength of this approach is that managers have the best knowledge available for forecasting – current working practices, technology used and performance levels that can be achieved.

However, the total level of projected staff requirements may then exceed what the organization as a whole can afford in the forecast period. The following possible weaknesses on the part of managers contribute to this problem.

1 Instead of deriving unit objectives from organizational goals, local interests and preferences may guide their assessments.
2 Local managers may be so entrenched in existing practices and procedures that ways of obtaining productivity increases are not identified and technological developments are overlooked.
3 Where units are not directly connected with service delivery, such as general administrative and support staff, the managers responsible have difficulty assessing staffing levels that reflect realistic average standards of performance. They tend to use subjective measures that, over time, allow staffing levels to rise gradually without any systematic analysis and justification. This is 'Parkinson's Law': that work expands to fill the time allowed for it. This can also happen when an organization is contracting its output. The tendency then is to adjust line staff to reduced levels of output, without reducing administrative and support staffing levels.
4 Local managers tend to overstate their requirements for staff for contingency purposes such as meeting peaks in output demand.

The top-down approach

Organizations have responded to these problems by adopting a top-down approach that, at its strongest, forecasts staffing requirements by specialists who report directly to the centre with a minimum involvement of line managers. These forecasts then conform to what senior management wants, in terms of expenditure targets in a given period. Sometimes, however, budget constraints are perceived as more severe than they really are, and output is then constrained by staffing shortages or gaps. The greatest weakness of this centralized approach is the lack of involvement by line managers, and consequently a failure to obtain their commitment to the plans adopted.

In order to prevent conflicts of interest shown by the top-down versus bottom-up arguments, top management usually compromises and allows a combination of both approaches to produce a demand forecast. Managers have a degree of freedom in contributing their own views to the aggregated forecast, but then have to adjust to meet the requirements of top management.

A more satisfactory way to resolve the bottom-up versus top-down dilemma is to prepare and agree criteria for demand forecasting that are affordable. Examples of criteria for reconciling staffing forecasts and resource availability are:

• administrative staff costs not to exceed 6 per cent of total staff costs;
• staff costs not to exceed targets set in line with economic growth or inflation rates.

To make this work, managers may need a planning cycle that enables participation at key decision points, and builds commitment towards a common interest in meeting organizational needs.

Case study: forecast of child health care assistants

The following fictional case study gives an example for a practical application of the indicator method of forecasting. In Delta Region, a Seventh National Five-Year Development Plan, commencing 1 January of Year 2, incorporates a proposal from the Ministry of Health to improve the health care of very young children.

The scheme involves the creation of a new post of Child Health Assistant, whose function is to provide regular health care for all children aged 3 years and under. Resources have been allocated for the recruitment, training and salary costs of the new group of health workers.

Delta Region was chosen for pilot implementation of the scheme because surveys show that it has the highest incidence of child mortality of any region in the country. A recent survey estimates the following mortality rates in the Delta Region:

under 1 year of age	12 per cent of live births
1 and under 2 years of age	3 per cent of those reaching the age of 1
2 and under 3 years of age	1 per cent of those reaching the age of 2

The National Census produced an estimate of the population of Delta Region of 2,481,000 on 1 January of Year 1. Preliminary comparisons between that census and the previous one (five years earlier) show that in Delta Region the total population increased by 2.9 per cent per annum between the two census years and the crude birth rate, that is the number of live births per 1000 of the population per year, remained unchanged at 44 during the period between the two census years. The Chief Census Officer advises that both these figures can be used for forecasting over the next four years (Years 2, 3, 4, 5).

A well-established health care scheme for young children in a neighbouring country, similar to that proposed, suggests that each Child Health Assistant can handle, on average, 3000 registered children aged 3 and under. The Chief Medical Officer of the Ministry of Health recommends that this figure should be incorporated in initial planning of the new scheme in Delta Region.

It is intended that the Child Health Scheme should become fully operational in Delta Region from 1 January of Year 5. This timescale allows three full years (2, 3, 4) for detailed service planning and training the new staff required.

Activity 8.4

Forecast the number of Child Health Assistant posts required in Delta Region on 1 January of Year 5. Assume that total forecast births in Year 5 are to be taken account of in the forecast. Start with the population forecast and then work out the number of live births for each year. Calculate then the number of children reaching the age of 1, 2 and 3 years in Years 3–5. Use Table 8.2 to undertake the forecast.

Table 8.2 Forecast of child health assistants: working sheet

year	population forecast, 1 January	live births forecast	number of children reaching the age of 1	number of children reaching the age of 2	number of children reaching the age of 3	total children in scheme, 1 January year 5
1						
2						
3						
4						
5						

↻ Feedback

Your table should look like Table 8.3:

Table 8.3 Forecast of child health assistants (completed)

year	population forecast, 1 January 9×1.0290	live births forecast (44×100)	number of children reaching the age of 1 (survival factor 0.88)	number of children reaching the age of 2 (survival factor 0.97)	number of children reaching the age of 3 (survival factor 0.99)	total children in scheme, 1 January year 5
1	2,481,000					
2	2,552,949	112,328				
3	2,626,985	115,588	98,849			
4	2,703,167	118,941	101,717	95,884		
5	2,781,559	122,390	104,668	98,665	94,925	420,648

Forecast number of Child Health Assistant posts Year 5:

$$\frac{420\,648}{3000} = 141.$$

Forecasting supply

Referring to the strategic framework in Figure 8.1, a supply analysis draws on a number of information components. The number of staff likely to be needed in a future time period requires knowing:

- the impact of current personnel policies on the capabilities and motivations of the workforce (Box 3);
- the details of current staff (Box 4); and
- the influence of the labour market on staff supply (Box 5).

The need for a personnel inventory

A personnel inventory lists all staff in an organization according to basic employment variables such as occupation, grade, department, age, length of service, qualifications and gender. Supply forecasting relies on being able to *aggregate* data from the personnel inventory, such as the number of staff in an occupational group and number of leavers in a year. Tables can then be constructed to show changes in total staff employed by category, age structure, male/female ratio and so on over relevant time periods. Computerized personnel information systems greatly ease the task of inventory compilation. Manual systems require much time-consuming clerical effort to extract data from individual records for an inventory. Visual presentation can aid managers' decision-making by facilitating agreement on problems and their further analysis. Trends and averages can be identified which highlight emergent human resource problems and opportunities faced by the organization.

Staff turnover and stability

An important use for the inventory is to establish trends in staff *wastage* from the organization, categorized according to avoidable reasons for leaving (such as wages or relationships between fellow workers) and unavoidable reasons (such as retirement).

The *turnover rate* is often used to measure wastage, particularly if trends are to be presented. In addition, or alternatively, the *stability index* can be used to measure how well a staff category is standing up to erosion in its numbers due to wastage from the organization. The turnover rate is usually calculated at year-end to summarize staff wastage during the year.

Turnover rate = (number of leavers in the year/ average number of staff employed in the year) × 100

The turnover rate can be misleading. Consider, for example, three similar departments that employ 100 employees.

1 Department A loses every employee at the beginning of the year and each is replaced by someone who stays until the following year.
2 Department B loses half its employees at the beginning of the year and their replacements also leave before the end of the year, hence need replacing.

3 Department C loses only four employees at the beginning of the year but their jobs are filled by a succession of people, each of whom stays only two weeks.

In each case, the turnover is 100 per cent. However, department A has lost all its skilled staff, department B has lost only half, and department C has lost only four. To present a more realistic picture of staff wastage, an alternative measure, the stability index, can be used.

Stability index = (number of staff with one year's service or more/ number of staff at start of year) × 100

 Activity 8.5

From the following information, calculate the turnover rate and the stability index for a hospital with 400 nurses.

Nurses at start of year	400
Leavers during year	45
Recruits during year	35
Net change of staff	(−) 10
Staff at year end	390

Feedback

The average number of nurses employed during year was 400 + 390 / 2 = 395

Staff with one year's service or more was 400 − 45 = 355

Turnover rate = (45/395) × 100 = 11.4 per cent

Stability index = (355/400) × 100 = 88.8 per cent

The importance of the external labour market

Personnel strategies that include recruiting skilled staff to bridge the gap between demand and supply invariably take account of the labour market. Important factors are:

- unemployment levels;
- degree of competition for staff with other employers in the area;
- output of people from the education system – schools and technical colleges – and the basic qualifications/skills likely to be available;
- local transport facilities;
- local housing schemes at appropriate prices/rents.

In addition, some national factors may affect the local situation over time:

- population movement related to the distribution of income/job opportunities;
- effects of government legislation, particularly on employment conditions;
- impact of development planning, particularly the location of economic zones of special opportunity;
- government training schemes, particularly those related to key skills provision.

It may be necessary to institute regular monitoring of aspects of the labour market likely to be significant for the organization in the future. Early identification of constraints on recruiting enough staff with key skills can stimulate ideas about alternative personnel strategies before serious problems arise – in short, anticipatory and proactive strategies.

Analysing the performance of human resource plans

During the implementation of human resource plans, data are collected and analysed for monitoring progress and assessing whether corrective action is necessary. This is done at two distinct levels:

Operational management This involves on the spot progress reviews to ensure that targets, including budgetary ones, are met by individuals and work teams. Immediate feedback to those concerned ensures corrective actions when necessary.

Strategic review This involves senior management in assessing the progress of operational plans according to a few key indicators directly related to organizational goals and objectives.

The 'usefulness' of human resource planning: choices facing organizations

At the beginning of this chapter, methods of precedence, analogy and individual managerial judgement were examined. HRP is about moving beyond such customary methods when they are no longer adequate to attune staff to strategic and budgetary needs, to overcome skill shortages, and provide an effective working environment.

Once the principle of planning is adopted, how should its scope and method be decided? One response is that a planning approach should be developed as long as it adds value to personnel decisions, but this is not easy to assess as no objective measure exists. Another response is to say that HRP is appropriate for *large and stable* health care organizations, which can better afford the employment of specialist human resource staff and other costs associated with it. However, it will still require managers to learn the concepts and techniques of HRP, and the money and time this requires may be a disincentive. In short, managers have to be convinced of the value of planning before they will support it.

What are the particular difficulties with HRP in the health sector?

There may be difficulties in measuring the output and quality of many services provided, and matching output to the contributions of different staff groups in the organization. The traditional hierarchy of command in the professional tiers often adds to these difficulties.

The difficulties of specifying purely quantitative measures of performance is another problem in health services. Quantitative measures (the numbers of patients treated, for example) say little about the quality in terms of effectiveness and efficiency.

Summary

You have learnt about a conceptual framework for HRP and the different activities necessary to the planning process including investigating; forecasting; planning; implementing; monitoring and evaluating. You have seen how HRP decisions can be taken on the basis of preceding staffing patterns, by analogy to other organizational units or by managerial judgement. You saw how demand forecasting methods related to performance indicators and assessed possible ways of reconciling a top-down with a bottom-up approach in HRP. You also examined models of assessing flows and stocks of staff, and discussed the application of staff turnover and stability indices. Finally, you saw the influence of the labour market on staff supply and some limitations of applying HRP in health care organizations.

References

Brahman, M. (1988) *Practical Manpower Planning*. London: Institute of Personnel Management.
Strike, A. (1995) *Human Resources in Health Care: A Manager's Guide*. Oxford: Blackwell Science.
Vickers, T. (1965) *The Art of Judgement*. London: Chapman Hall.

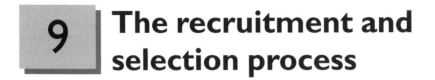

9 The recruitment and selection process

Overview

This chapter gives you an overview of staff recruitment and selection in health systems and develops a model of good practice. You will explore the obstacles to implementing the good practice model in the context of health care organizations and examine issues related to equal opportunities and the avoidance of discrimination. Finally, a variety of options for recruiting and filling staff vacancies is considered.

Learning objectives

After working through this chapter you will be able to:

- **apply a good practice model to the process of recruitment and selection;**
- **describe methods and techniques used in the selection process;**
- **outline limitations to the good practice model;**
- **understand different methods for filling staff vacancies;**
- **identify the types of discriminatory practices that can operate in recruitment and selection; and**
- **propose measures to combat discrimination and promote equal opportunities.**

Key terms

Assessment centre approach An approach to filling a staff post that combines several selection methods.

Discrimination The tendency to give preference to one social group, disregarding the merits of the other groups (for example, men over women).

Favouritism The tendency to ignore considerations of merit by giving preference to members of one's own family, ethnic group or geographical region, or to individuals favoured for some other personal reason.

Job description A description of the job, including its main purpose, responsibilities and key tasks.

Nepotism The granting of special consideration to members of one's own family.

Person specification An outline of the abilities, qualifications and experience required of the job-holder, usually distinguishing between essential and desirable requirements.

Positive action The inclusion of a positive statement of non-discrimination in advertising for applicants, or providing special arrangements such as flexi-time, nurseries or job-sharing for workers with young children.

Positive discrimination Selection that favours people from a disadvantaged group.

Stakeholders Those involved in a selection process who can affect, or are affected by, the appointment.

Training specification An account of the knowledge and skills (technical and social) the post-holder needs to perform the job satisfactorily.

Key stages in the recruitment and selection process

There are eight stages to the recruitment and selection of staff. These stages can be summarized as follows:

1 Job description
2 Person specification
3 Advertisement
4 Further particulars
5 Shortlisting
6 Interview
7 References
8 Final decision

The job description

The starting point in recruitment and selection is the development of a *job description*. This details the duties which prospective staff must carry out. Table 9.1 is an example of a job description for the post of Personnel Officer in a Tanzanian local authority. As you study it, note that the format is straightforward and that a standard format has been used.

The person specification

The second stage is the *person specification*. Table 9.2 is an example of a person specification for the same post. It is based on the job description and was obtained by editing the replies of relevant staff who were asked what skills, experience and knowledge would be needed to carry out each of the duties of the job description. Note that only a limited number of separate items should be listed. This is because selection at later stages in the process becomes unwieldy if there are too many items.

It is important to distinguish between *essential* and *desirable* requirements for the job. An essential requirement is one without which the post-holder would be unable to do the job. Examples are professional qualifications for doctors and nurses, but it could also be the ability to travel around the area in which the post is

Table 9.1 An example of a typical job description

Job title	Personnel Officer		
Post number	164	**Grade**	GS2
Department	Personnel and Administration	**Location**	Council Headquarters
Responsible to	Principal Manpower Management Officer		
Staff responsible for	Registry assistants		
Job purpose	(The main objectives to be achieved by the post-holder)		
	1 Advise officers and councillors in all personnel matters.		
	2 Carry out a full range of personnel duties.		
	3 Ensure that up-to-date information about the local authority's staff is available at all times.		
Main activities	(What the post-holder will actually do; what prescribed duties the post-holder will have)		
	1 Prepare and maintain personnel files continuously.		
	2 Prepare personnel emoluments (annual).		
	3 Counsel staff who have personal problems as required.		
	4 Continuously update personal knowledge of LGSC staff regulations and interpret them to staff and councillors as required.		
	5 Recruit and select staff up to GS4 as required.		
	6 Implement disciplinary procedure as required.		
	7 Coordinate performance appraisal for the council as a whole and implement appraisal for staff in the Personnel and Administration Department (annual).		
	8 Prepare and implement a training programme (annual).		
	9 Prepare minutes of management team meetings as required.		
	10 Any other duties which are within the scope of this appointment and which are requested by the Executive Director.		
Form prepared by	M Njunwa	**Date**	15.1.05

located – a hygiene inspector who has to visit several facilities, for example. A desirable requirement is one that contributes to effective performance but which is not essential. This could be a certain amount of work experience. You should avoid listing requirements as essential if they are not strictly so. There is a real danger of discrimination here and this will be considered later in the chapter.

Advertising

The third stage in the selection process is the advertisement. You are likely to be familiar with this stage: the newspaper advertisement, the notice on the organization notice-board, or the website on the Internet. Those who make enquiries in response to the advertisement will receive some written material, often described as the *further particulars* of the post. This material normally includes an application form, the job description and the person specification. It may also include information about the organization, the department in which the job is located and other information relevant to the needs of applicants.

Table 9.2 An example of a person specification

Post	Personnel Officer	
Grade	MMO2	
Attribute		Essential (E) or Desirable (D)
Skills		
Communication skills		E
Counselling skills		E
Administrative skills		E
Experience		
Three years' experience of administrative duties		D
Experience of local government work		D
Experience of personnel work		D
Knowledge		
(includes required qualifications, if any)		
Advanced Diploma in Public Administration or degree or equivalent		E
Knowledge of the schemes of service		D
Knowledge of the local community		D
Special requirements		
Age 18–45		E
Able to satisfy medical requirements		E
Prepared by	Sola, N	
Authorized by	Njunwa, M	
Date	15 December 2005	

Shortlisting applicants

When selecting applicants for a job, often a *selection panel* is used for *shortlisting* using the selection criteria of the person specification for the post. The procedure is used to filter out candidates who do not fit the person specification and to select from the remainder those to be invited to the *final selection stage*. The final selection stage may comprise a number of different elements, of which the one probably most familiar to you is the *selection interview*. However, where there are many potentially suitable applicants (for example, to work in support services in large organizations), applicants may be asked to sit a qualifying test or to write a short report – in other words, something to demonstrate whether they have the skills for the job.

Appointing staff

Following selection, the organization is in a position to make an appointment. Before the appointment is confirmed, organizations normally ask candidates to nominate reliable informants who can provide an opinion in writing – usually called a *reference*, or testimonial – based on their personal knowledge about the candidate's suitability for the post. Organizations typically take up references either when the candidates are invited to the final selection stage, or following the final selection stage for the candidate recommended for appointment.

Issues of staff selection

Labour market conditions

In Chapter 8 you were introduced to the concept of the labour market in terms of its *supply* side, consisting of job-seekers and the abilities they offer; and the *demand* side, consisting of employers who wish to use those abilities. As with any market, the labour market may be loose or tight. In a *loose labour market*, there is a large number of job-seekers in competition for a small number of jobs and the employer can afford to pick and choose (a buyer's market). In a *tight labour market*, there is a small number of job-seekers available to fill a large number of jobs, and any employer, in competition with other employers, needs to make an effort to attract suitable workers (a seller's market).

Whilst a labour market may be generally loose or tight, there are likely to be areas where skilled staff are scarce – for example, for medical specialists. Alternatively, there might be geographical areas, such as remote areas or areas with an unfavourable climate, where job-seekers are unwilling to reside and work, despite the relative availability of jobs.

Activity 9.1

Taking the labour market for nurses in your country as an example:

1   Would you describe it as generally loose or tight at the moment?
2   In what skill areas or geographical areas, relevant to health services, is the market relatively tight?
3   What measures might be used to loosen those areas of tightness?

Feedback

There are a number of incentives employers can use to improve labour market conditions, such as better pay and working conditions, flexible working hours for women, allowances for rural areas. The approach that an employer takes to attracting candidates will vary in line with labour market conditions. Often public sector organizations are not sufficiently sensitive to those conditions. They may continue to assume that they will have a steady stream of nurses, say, even when working conditions in public hospitals are deteriorating and staff find better paid positions in the private sector. Owing to resource shortages in the health sector there may be also an inability of the national labour market to absorb all medical and nursing graduates, causing migration of skilled health workers.

The following measures by employers in Singapore to deal with the problem of labour shortage provide a good example (Torrington and Hunt, 1994). The policies are similar to those countries which have attracted migrant health workers in the past – for example, Asian doctors to work as GPs in Britain during the 1960s, Korean nurses working in Germany in the 1970s, Bangladeshi nurses to the Gulf states, or foreign medical graduates in the USA in the 1990s and 2000s.

Case example: a response to demographic change in Singapore

In Singapore in the 1990s, changes in demographic and labour supply factors caused a tightening of labour markets. Similar problems were encountered in several other South-East Asian countries, especially in those locations where economic development had been very rapid.

- *Recruiting foreign workers*: Singapore employers are responding to the current labour shortage by hiring foreign workers who have been attracted to Singapore because of the high pay. However, their attempts to recruit more foreign workers is constrained by the Ministry of Labour, which imposes a foreign worker levy as well as a quota based on a local–foreigner ratio. In recent years, Malaysian employers have also become increasingly dependent on foreign workers, especially those from neighbouring Indonesia. Recently, the Malaysian government has also introduced a foreign worker levy on employers.
- *Intensifying recruitment efforts* through advertising campaigns and posters, liaising with employment agents in neighbouring countries.
- *Strengthening liaison with schools and polytechnics* by participating in industrial attachment schemes and providing work experience opportunities for students.
- *Enhancing career development*: in order to retain existing workers, many employers are now paying attention to better training facilities; job restructuring/ multi-skilling; career development programmes; better promotion prospects; employee participation through quality improvement activities.
- *Women*: in order to attract more female workers, some Singapore employers are experimenting with flexible hours as well as part-time work. A problem facing many employers is the lack of child care facilities. Many Singaporean women have left the labour market after childbirth because of the lack of suitable child care facilities. Whilst the highly paid female professionals can afford to employ maids to help them with household chores and child care, their lower-paid counterparts in the factories prefer to stay at home with their children.
- *Older workers*: in view of the labour shortage, some Singaporean employers have extended the present retirement age from 55 to 60. Some have introduced flexible retirement arrangements to retain their older employees.
- *Students*: some companies employ students on a part-time basis to overcome their labour shortage problem. This has become a common phenomenon in restaurants, fast food and retail outlets.

Alternative shortlisting method – rating applicants

A common mistake in shortlisting is to pay too much attention to the presentation of the application at the expense of its content. This is especially true when there is no guidance on how to carry out shortlisting and people rely on their own intuitions about what makes someone a good employee. For example, in a study of decision processes in the assessment of job application forms in six organizations (two each in transport, computer and manufacturing companies), it was found that one in five comments related to presentation rather than job-related ability (Herriot and Wingrove, 1984).

Developing *decision aids* can enable recruiters to rate applicants according to their capabilities and remove some of the bias that otherwise may be involved. The decision aid usually involves some form of *scoring scheme* in which each of the selection criteria identified in the person specification is scored, say, from 1 to 10.

Whilst scoring is an effective procedure in shortlisting candidates, it has to be implemented with due care. For example, if a scaled system is used, selectors should try to use the full length of the scoring scale: they should be ready to award 0 out of 10, or 10 out of 10, if the candidate deserves it, rather than just clustering their scores within a narrower range. Selectors should also try to mark each criterion separately, rather than mark on their general feeling about the candidate. With each criterion they should ask 'What evidence have we got of the candidate's ability in this area?', and base their score on that evidence. Finally, if more than one selector is involved in shortlisting (which is desirable to counteract individual bias), they should score independently. If the selectors then go on to discuss scores, they should not be swayed by any special pleading on the part of the other selector.

When shortlisting is done effectively using scoring methods, the decision about whom to invite to interview is straightforward: you simply sum selectors' scores, and the highest-scoring candidates are invited to interview. A record of the scores should be retained as evidence of how the organization accepted or rejected certain candidates. This will be valuable if the selection decision is challenged by an unsuccessful candidate, either through an organization's internal grievance procedure or through a court of law. This is very common in many countries, and a written record of good practice procedure helps a successful defence against such challenges.

Inviting candidates in the selection stage

Candidates who have been shortlisted will be invited formally to attend a final selection stage. *Transparency* of the selection process is an important management principle at this stage. It is good practice that candidates should receive as much information as possible about how selection is managed and how the organization will reach its decision. If, for example, there is going to be a test, candidates should be briefed on what kind of test it will be. If there is going to be a panel interview, candidates should be informed approximately how long it will last, and who the members of the panel will be. There is a civil liberties argument in favour of transparency: that candidates, who provide confidential information about themselves, should know how the organization will use that confidential information.

The interview is the most widely used *and* the most heavily criticized of all final selection methods. You have most probably taken part in one, either as selector or candidate. An interview is sometimes defined as 'a conversation with a purpose'. It is a meeting, usually lasting anything from five minutes to one hour, between a representative or representatives of the employer who asks questions, and a candidate who has to answer them – though she or he may be allowed to ask a few questions too.

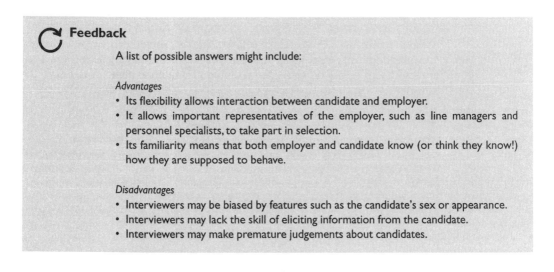

Activity 9.2

Drawing on your own experiences, make a short list of the advantages and disadvantages of the selection interview.

Feedback

A list of possible answers might include:

Advantages
- Its flexibility allows interaction between candidate and employer.
- It allows important representatives of the employer, such as line managers and personnel specialists, to take part in selection.
- Its familiarity means that both employer and candidate know (or think they know!) how they are supposed to behave.

Disadvantages
- Interviewers may be biased by features such as the candidate's sex or appearance.
- Interviewers may lack the skill of eliciting information from the candidate.
- Interviewers may make premature judgements about candidates.

The assessment centre approach to selection

A basic principle of selection is gaining enough evidence on the range of skills a candidate has as regards each element of the person specification. Table 9.3 illustrates a *selection grid* designed to provide the evidence you need to select, for example, a personnel manager for a district hospital.

The left-hand column lists the selection criteria whilst the other columns represent four methods of obtaining good evidence for each criterion. There are two important principles at work in the selection grid shown:

- There should be at least two separate sources of evidence for each major criterion (evidence is inevitably conditioned by the method used to obtain it; therefore it is desirable to have more than one method or source).
- The design should be able to yield evidence for more than one criterion.

Table 9.3 Selection grid

Criterion	Form	Interview	Written test	Presentation
Counselling skills		✓		✓
Report-writing ability	✓		✓	
Presentation skills		✓		✓
Experience of personnel work	✓	✓		✓
Knowledge of hospital administration	✓	✓	✓	
Advanced diploma or degree	✓			

In Table 9.3 there are two sources for each criterion, with the exception of 'advanced diploma or degree', for which the application should provide adequate evidence. In the case of the second principle, each method provides evidence for at least two criteria. Thus the table conforms to the two principles stated.

This approach to selection is called an *assessment centre* approach. Notice the role of the interview in this process: rather than acting as the only method of final selection, it is but one element or method, amongst others, in the selection procedure. Like other elements, it is used to obtain evidence for specific criteria; it is not used to provide a final summary judgement on candidates. In practical terms, these methods can be employed alongside each other at the final selection. Thus one candidate might be giving a presentation whilst another is attending the interview, and so on. Following the completion of all the elements, a review session is held in which evidence obtained by different methods is pooled and a final decision made.

Written tests and presentations are two examples of assessment centre activities which are widely used. Other methods include various group activities: candidates as a group may be given a problem to solve or may be asked to attend a meeting in which each candidate is given a specific role to play, perhaps to argue a particular point of view on an issue. Such activities provide evidence of *interpersonal skills* and *problem-solving ability*. A further method is the 'in-basket exercise': candidates are asked to deal with a series of items which represent the work of the post for which they are being considered. Such an activity provides evidence of ability to *organize a workload* and of *analytical skills*. Research suggests that the assessment centre approach is highly effective in selecting the right candidates.

Using tests in selection

Recognition of the limitations of the interview has led to the development of other selection methods, especially the *ability test*. Some advantages of commercially available tests are:

- They have gone through a rigorous process of test development, so that the test results are highly reliable.
- They are accompanied by test manuals which give explicit instructions on how the tests should be used – and also on how they should not be used.
- The more recent tests contain information about the relative performance of women and men, which the selector can use to help interpret test results and avoid discrimination.

There are also some disadvantages:

- Published tests are expensive and are only available in countries where the test agencies have representatives.
- Access to the published test is restricted to staff who have received specialist training, which again is expensive.
- Tests are seen as threatening by many candidates and insulting by others. Research suggests, for instance, that tests that are accepted as normal by German or British candidates may be resented by French or Italian candidates, because tests are used much less frequently in these countries.

Limitations of the good practice model

The stages of recruitment and selection described above are widely regarded as good practice. However, most surveys of selection practices in organizations in the United States and Europe consistently show that the best methods are not the most widely used. There are two main reasons for this. First, the best practice model requires considerable resources of time and money: a two-day assessment centre, for example, will use plenty of both.

Second, and more subtly, introducing this model of good practice may disturb the balance of power in an organization. In the absence of a properly designed and integrated selection process, selection is undertaken, as often as not, by senior members of staff who exercise a great deal of discretion in appointing the candidates they favour. In this situation, introducing a systematic approach limits managers' freedom of discretion and may also represent a transfer of power over appointments from the line manager to the human resource specialist.

✎ Activity 9.3

Suppose you want to fill the post of the leading paediatrician in a hospital. Who are the stakeholders likely to be in your country?

↻ Feedback

Compare your answer with the one shown in Figure 9.1. This is what is sometimes called a stakeholder map. It is a visual method of identifying the stakeholders who have an interest in an appointment (or, for that matter, who have an interest in any organizational decision).

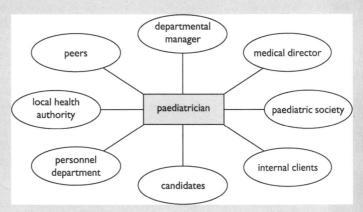

Figure 9.1 Example of a stakeholder map

Source: Adapted from Freeman (1984).

It is important to recognize, therefore, that different *stakeholders* may have different, indeed competing, interests in the selection of staff. The character of the stakeholders may vary from one organization to another. For example, there may be local politicians, employee representation, unions, board members of the hospital, and even members of the public who have pressurized for the new post. It is not enough, therefore, to choose the most sophisticated selection method. You must tailor your choice to the character of the different stakeholders involved. In general, it is better to use a method which is less sophisticated if the stakeholders will be more committed to the appointment. As in other areas of management, the good practice solution which appears to be the most rational or the most technically sound is not always the best one.

Other methods of filling staff vacancies

Not all vacant positions in an organization require the time-consuming task of a selection and recruitment process. Here are five other methods (there may be others).

Reallocation of duties

When a post becomes vacant because of a departure of a member of staff, you may prefer simply to spread the duties of the post amongst other staff in the same unit. Perhaps changes in the work of the unit mean that some of the duties of the post are no longer carried out. Perhaps there is a freeze on recruitment, which means that the manager simply will not get permission to recruit and must therefore do the best he or she can.

Transfer of posts

Many posts are filled by transfer rather than as a result of recruitment and selection. For instance, hospitals may have graduate development or other staff development programmes. That means that certain posts are earmarked to be filled on a temporary basis by an employee who is on such a development programme.

Redeployment

Health care organizations that need to reduce posts often seek to redeploy redundant staff in another unit. Thus a line manager will be asked to accept someone from a redeployment pool as an alternative to advertising a vacancy in the normal way.

Outsourcing

An aspect of new public management is the contracting-out of public services. For example, catering and cleaning services may be carried out by a private firm contracted to the health care organization responsible for the service. Even whole clinical departments can be contracted out to the private sector. The same thing is frequently done with individual posts. Thus, a hospital may find it cheaper to use an agency to recruit nurses than to fill the post in the normal way. Of course, this also allows the manager to hire temporary staff without having to go through lengthy administrative procedures.

Appointment of a previously identified successor

Some organizations may have formal succession planning programmes, where a deputy is identified who will automatically step into a post – usually a very senior post – when its incumbent retires or comes to the end of his or her contract. Such successor arrangements are suitable where the post is unique to the organization and where skills needed to do it can only be gained in the organization. This is an option rarely used in health services, but it is sometimes used in the succession of the board of hospital directors.

Case study: identifying and selecting staff options

Wellville has too many hospital beds in relation to its population and funding agencies are demanding a reduction. One out of the five public hospitals in Wellville has recently been closed; the remaining four are now coming under increasing pressure to improve efficiency and to reduce capacity. This has had an impact on staffing decisions in three ways.

Pressure to cut staff costs – a redundancy programme has started. Although most of the redundancies so far have been voluntary, some compulsory redundancies have been made in areas such as catering where outside contractors are beginning to be used.

Redeployment – some staff have been offered redeployment as an alternative to redundancy, and a central redeployment pool has been established.

Need to justify decisions to recruit – line managers are expected to provide a convincing justification for the recruitment of new staff, although top management has recognized that there are some priority areas of activity which should be protected. For instance, there is a great deal of concern about standards of maintenance of the buildings.

The programme of reconstructing wards in two of the hospitals was disrupted by the recent financial crisis and there was major uncertainty about future investment in the hospitals. However a recent government decision has protected spending on the maintenance programme, ensuring competitiveness with the private sector.

Another area which might also be regarded as a priority is the nursing training centre. Government has signalled a commitment to nursing training, as the unit is the only one providing continuous training for hospital nurses in the region. The staff training unit has recently been delegated a great deal of financial control, including control of the unit's staffing budget.

The unit now has a vacancy for a training officer, created by the retirement of a very experienced member of staff. That person had been responsible for a long-established programme of supervisory training, which has been declining in demand during the shrinking of the hospital sector in the last three years.

Activity 9.4

Having read this case study write a brief report that:

1 outlines the staffing options (recruitment and alternatives) available to the staff training unit;
2 presents an argument to support your preferred option.

Feedback

Some of the advantages and disadvantages of the various options have been set out in Table 9.4. Compare the points listed there with the points that you have made in your own answer.

Which of the options is preferable? You can certainly rule out a couple of them. The last option, appointment of a successor, is not applicable since no successor has been identified. The first option, simply appointing a replacement, seems foolish because it is known that the demand for the supervisory training for which the

Table 9.4 Advantages and disadvantages of staffing options

Staffing option	Advantages	Disadvantages
Recruitment of a replacement	allows unit to draw on skills in the labour market	confines post to training for which demand is reducing
Reallocation of duties	allows declining demand for supervisory training to be met by existing staff; may release post for new work	may overload existing staff; union or staff representatives may object
Transfer	facilitates development of existing member of staff	transferee may not have relevant skills
Redeployment of a supernumerary	prevents member of staff being made redundant	supernumerary may not have relevant skills
Outsourcing	unit's control of staffing budget makes this possible; would enable commitment to supervisory training to be met flexibly as demand reduces	suitable consultant may not be available; union or staff representatives may object
Appointment of a previously identified successor	not applicable – no successor has been identified	not applicable

retiring training officer has been responsible is reducing. Moreover, such an appointment would be difficult to justify. Amongst the other options, your preference will depend on the point of view from which you approach this. Government responsibility for all hospitals in Wellville will want the training unit to consider redeployment and may have someone whom they would like to transfer as part of a development programme. The staff training unit itself will probably be keener to outsource or to reallocate duties, since that would release money which the unit can use for other purposes.

Discriminatory practices in recruitment and selection

Applying good practice is particularly appropriate to confront problems of discrimination, nepotism and favouritism.

- *Discrimination* is the tendency to give preference to one social group and to disregard the merits of other groups.
- *Nepotism* or *favouritism* is the tendency to ignore considerations of merit by giving preference to members of one's own family, ethnic group or geographical region, or to individuals who are favoured for some other personal reason (because they support the same political party, for example, or because they have offered a bribe).

A cartoon (Figure 9.2) appeared in *The Herald*, a Zimbabwean newspaper, in 1985, and suggests three ways in which appointments (and promotions) were made. The practices of nepotism, favouritism and discrimination in employment are so prevalent in many countries that you should spend a little time considering them before seeing how good practice can contribute to limiting their force.

Corruption

Corruption in health services has many different faces, such as the following.

1 At the interface between the medical–industrial complex and health workers:
   - corruption of the medical literature where authors fail to disclose a conflict of interest and are being paid by an industry to produce results in favour of their products (e.g. pharmaceuticals, tobacco, asbestos);
   - bribing of officials to approve new drugs;
   - excessive pricing of medical supplies, articles and sharing profits between the supply company and the health care professional;
   - institutionalized corruption in the form of travel scholarships, meetings, rebates granted by the industry;
   - fake prescriptions reimbursed by insurance companies or ghost deliveries of drugs to health centres, or distribution of expired drugs.

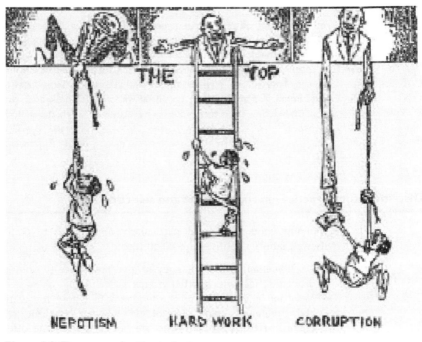

Figure 9.2 Three ways of getting to the top
Source: *The Herald*, Zimbabwe, 1985

2   At the interface between staff and patients:

- 'unofficial' user fees where incentives for output are lacking or health professionals are poorly paid;
- 'under-the-table money' as part of the doctor's fee.

All these forms of corruption impinge on human resources as they affect the power distribution in organizations and involve additional cost to the user. Of course, there is a range of views on corruption and there are cultural differences in the acceptance of these practices. Sometimes corruption is seen as just oiling the wheels or, in economic terms, as enhancing efficiency by giving officials a quasi-price incentive to work (Weiner, 1962). However, in real terms the costs of corruption add substantially to the costs of health care which the individual and society have to bear.

In Robert Wade's (1989) book on doctors in India, corruption was seen to have become *institutionalized*, to the extent that the price paid for different jobs was semi-public knowledge. Although he suggested possible areas for reform, a pessimistic impression was created of the difficulties of fighting corruption that is so thoroughly entrenched.

Ethnic and sex discrimination

Favouritism can take many specific forms, such as the favouring of one ethnic group over another, which is called *ethnic* (or race) *discrimination*, or of men over women, *sex discrimination*. Britain has a long history of both kinds of discrimination. For example, in 1977 David Smith revealed how Asian and West Indian applicants for white-collar jobs faced discrimination in 30 per cent of cases, whilst there were significant differences in levels of discrimination between different types of jobs, and between men's and women's experience. Smith argued that the social structure from within which people's attitudes are formed should be changed. In Britain, his work contributed to the development of the Race Relations and Sex Discrimination Act, the principles of which have become socially and politically accepted.

Ask yourself this question: is discrimination on ethnic, sex or any other grounds a problem in your country?

Direct and indirect discrimination

There is a distinction between *direct* and *indirect* discrimination. Direct discrimination is a simple concept. In sex terms, it means directly favouring a man over a woman simply because he is a man, and for no other reason. Indirect discrimination is more subtle. It means applying a condition or requirement to both women and men which has a *disproportionate adverse impact* on women – that is, women find it harder to meet the requirement – and which cannot be justified in terms of the needs of the job. It is equally possible for a man to argue that a condition or requirement discriminates against him as a man *in exactly the same way* – even though in practice the incidence of discrimination against men is probably lower than discrimination against women in every country in the world.

So there is a two-stage test of indirect discrimination:

1 Does the condition or requirement have a disproportionate effect?
2 Is the condition or requirement justifiable in terms of the needs of the job?

For indirect discrimination to be present, the answer to the first question must be 'yes' and the answer to the second question must be 'no'. It is quite possible for a requirement to have disproportionate effects but still be justifiable. For instance, some manual jobs could have a requirement that staff need to be able to lift heavy weights. This would be harder for the average woman to comply with than for the average man. But the requirement would not be discriminatory as long as the employer could show that it was necessary in terms of the duties of the job. (Notice that this would not be a reason to exclude all women applicants. Some of them would be able to lift heavy weights, just as some men would not.)

Discrimination in the selection process

After discussing these problems of discrimination, you may now feel that selection is a minefield that public sector managers enter at their peril. Certainly, indirect discrimination is a subtle concept and many of the selection criteria which public agencies have used without question for many years may well turn out to be discriminatory on closer inspection.

Employers are most likely to discriminate by requiring particular paid work experience or a particular qualifications where experience shows that men are more likely than women to have those kinds of work experience and qualifications (and the same may be true where some ethnic groups are concerned). On the other hand, there is less difficulty in listing criteria under the headings of skills as essential, since individuals can acquire skills in different ways. For instance, management skills are necessary in many senior jobs. But while such skills can be gained through paid work experience or by study, they can be gained in other ways too.

Activity 9.5

Assume that you have recently launched an equal opportunity initiative in your health care organization but the proportion of disadvantaged members of society has not increased. Why, despite all efforts to eliminate discrimination, are more members of disadvantaged groups not being appointed? Assuming that discrimination has been eliminated (a difficult assumption to make!), what possible reasons do you think there could be for this state of affairs?

Feedback:

Some of the possible reasons are:

1 Even when only necessary job requirements are stated as essential, many members of disadvantaged groups still do not meet them.

2 Potential applicants, *believing* that discrimination continues, choose not to apply.

3 Even members of disadvantaged groups who are willing to apply and who meet the requirements are unable to satisfy the conditions of the job.

Overcoming disadvantage: demand-side intervention

There are a number of interventions that can be made by employers in their demand for recruits – through *positive discrimination, positive action* and *publicity*, and the provision of employee services to help overcome problems specific to the disadvantaged group. These are described below.

Positive discrimination

In this intervention, the employer decides to consider only members of the disadvantaged group for the next vacancy or to set a *quota* of vacancies that will be reserved for them. This is the practice that is sometimes called *positive dis-*

crimination. Where the problem of under-representation of certain groups is felt to be very great, public agencies may resort to positive discrimination. For example, in India and the United States there have been quotas for disadvantaged ethnic groups (which are known in India as 'scheduled castes') to enter higher education.

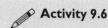
Activity 9.6

Such action may appear to be a simple solution. But can you see any difficulties?

Feedback

There appear to be at least four:

1 The action may be struck down in the law courts as being in breach of a specific law, or in breach of constitutional guarantees of equal treatment for all.

2 It may cause dissatisfaction amongst precisely those groups whom it was intended to benefit: members of the disadvantaged group may resent the implication that they were appointed because of their membership of that group, and not on merit.

3 It may simply not be possible: only qualified doctors can be appointed to a medical position, only qualified nurses to nursing positions, and so on.

4 For the public employer, it may conflict with the obligation to provide the best quality of service possible. Positive discrimination is only invoked, after all, when it seems preferable to appoint someone who is not in other ways the best person for the job.

Admittedly, there are instances where one might argue that only a member of a particular group can do the job effectively (this is termed a *genuine occupational qualification*). For instance, it seems reasonable that female nurses should care for female patients when there is a requirement for privacy.

Positive action and publicity

The problems of positive discrimination can be so great that other policies to encourage the employment of members of disadvantaged groups have been advocated. They are known as *positive action* to distinguish them from positive discrimination. Such action often involves *publicity* to persuade disadvantaged groups to apply for jobs by stating that employers will not discriminate against them. For example, many employers add the phrase 'We are an equal opportunity employer welcoming applications from all sections of the community' to their job advertisements.

Practical measures are also used to promote applications from those, particularly women, with other work and family duties. Very often, women stay at home whilst their children are young, returning to outside work only after they have started school. Even then, it is often the mother who is responsible for getting the children to school and collecting them at the end of the day. If working hours clash with school hours, the mother may be unable to work. There are a number of schemes to improve working conditions for women, some of which have been applied to health services:

- introducing 'flexi-time', so that staff can fix their own working hours, as long as they work the specified number of hours in a week; this allows parents, for example, to leave children at school on their way to work;
- setting up a workplace nursery, where parents can leave children below school age whilst they are working;
- introducing 'job-sharing', so that two members of staff can share a single job, enabling both to spend more time with their families;
- introducing a 'career break' scheme, so that staff with children have a period of leave without pay for up to three years whilst children are very young.

Notice that, with the exception of the nursery (for which parents themselves may have to pay), none of the above measures has a financial cost. Indeed, one can argue that there is an efficiency gain: in the case of job-share, for instance, the employers get two heads for the price of one.

Overcoming disadvantages: supply intervention

Even with the above measures (and putting aside positive discrimination), there may still be many members of disadvantaged groups who are not eligible to apply for public vacancies because they lack the required qualifications. For example, when Royal Nepal Airlines Corporation, the national airline of Nepal, advertised for aeronautical engineers in 1995, all the candidates who applied were male.

Historical patterns of disadvantage often mean that members of disadvantaged groups reach the point of selection without the necessary qualifications or experience. In such cases, public employers may provide special training targeted at the disadvantaged groups as a way of bridging the gap (this is sometimes called *positive action training*). Thus when the Local Government Service Commission in Tanzania organized professional training for senior personnel specialists working in local authorities, they set aside some places on the training courses for more junior personnel staff who were female so that they would be qualified for promotion to senior positions when posts became available later on.

Some countries have gone further than this, reserving places in higher education for members of disadvantaged groups, often through the operation of quotas. However, as has been stressed already, this is often a controversial policy and strong political support is needed to make it successful.

Summary

You have learnt how good practice model of recruitment and selection consists of a sequence of different elements. In the final decision stage, there may be a need to use a combination of selection methods in an assessment centre approach. The need to understand the different stakeholders in this process was examined and a variety of alternative staffing options available to health service managers reviewed. Finally, you saw how to combat favouritism, corruption and discrimination through structural change.

References

Freeman, R. E. (1984) *Strategic Management: A Stakeholder Approach*. Marshfield, Massachusetts: Pitman.

Herriot, P. and Wingrove, J. (1984) Decision process in graduate pre-selection, *Journal of Occupational Psychology*, 57: 269–75.

Smith, D. (1977) *Racial Discrimination in Britain*. Harmondsworth: Penguin.

Torrington, D. and Hunt, T. (1994) *Human Resource Management in South-East Asia*. Singapore: Prentice Hall.

Wade, R. (1989) Politics and graft: recruitment, appointment, and promotions to public office in India, in P. Ward (ed.) *Corruption, Development and Inequality*. London: Routledge, pp. 73–109.

Weiner, M. (1962) *The Policy of Scarcity: Public Press and Political Response in India*. Chicago: University of Chicago Press.

10 Performance management, appraisal and career development

Overview

In this chapter you will learn about performance management, appraisal and career development. The objective of performance management is to set targets for individual jobs and staff, in order to fulfil the organization's goals. You will also look at the problems of introducing and implementing appraisal systems in health care organizations.

Learning objectives

After working through this chapter you will be able to:

- **outline the approach of management by objectives (MBO) and its links with performance management;**
- **identify objectives of health care organizations and link them to the performance of individuals and teams;**
- **outline the key stages of staff appraisal;**
- **outline current concepts of career development and its links with performance appraisal;**
- **identify problems in introducing and implementing performance appraisal systems;**
- **identify the main criticisms of individual appraisal methods and outline how appraisal systems can be modified to assess teamwork.**

Key terms

Appraisal Assessment of the performance of personnel within an organization based on specified standards and procedures.

Appraisal interview A meeting between a member of staff (appraisee) and his or her appraiser, to discuss the appraisee's performance, expectations and prospects within the organization.

Career development The development of a staff member's career within the organization. The acquisition of skills and experience enabling employees to attain more senior positions within the organization.

Career paths The normal routes of progression within an organization. They provide a source of information for employees to make choices about personal advancement, and for the organization they provide a way of ensuring that jobs relate to strategic goals, by identifying the key attributes post-holders should possess and how those attributes should be developed.

> **Performance** The process of achieving aims both at the organizational level and with respect to contributions to those aims at the level of work units and individual staff.

The theoretical roots of performance management

Performance management has gained credence in recent years with both public and private sector managers. Current approaches have their roots in what is termed 'management by objectives' (MBO). One of its main exponents, Humble (1970), saw the approach as ideal for public sector organizations, in which it is hard to quantify and/or value outputs. Humble suggested that management by objectives can provide the necessary techniques and disciplines to achieve success. Performance management has inherited this underlying philosophy of linking goals to individual job contributions, using both quantitative and qualitative factors to measure levels of achievement.

Establishing a performance management system

A performance management system begins with objective setting by top management by answering the question 'What does the organization exist to do?'. Invariably, the answer reflects the political and financial context of the organization. Thus, in health services, the answer must take into consideration four major themes:

1 *Effectiveness* – the delivery of services according to set objectives, such as improvement of health in terms of quality of life and survival.
2 *Efficiency* – the production of health at minimum cost within a system that is transparent and with managerial accountability for expenditure.
3 *Equity* – the provision of equal access to all clients who can benefit from the service; the management of human resources in a non-discriminatory manner with respect to sex, race and other social factors.
4 *Humanity* – the acceptability of services measured in terms of patient satisfaction; managing human resources in a way that respects patients' autonomy and dignity.

Once organizational purpose is established, it has to be translated into required contributions at the level of departments and units, and then individual jobs. This requires a cascade analysis, on the basis of the following questions.

1 What are the critical success factors for the organization – the activities which must be done well if its overall purpose is to be achieved?
2 For each success factor, how near is/are the current outcome(s) to what is required?
3 What has to be done to close the gap between current outcome(s) and the level(s) required?
4 How can individual work units contribute to closing the gap between current and required outcomes?
5 What is the implication for individual jobs in terms of their key tasks?

The concept of key tasks is central to performance management and informs job descriptions and job plans. Reddin (1971) defines six key tasks which contribute to organizational effectiveness:

1   managing people
2   identifying new products/services/techniques
3   developing new products/services/techniques
4   reaching time, cost and quality standards in output/delivery
5   improving organizational systems
6   enhancing organizational collaboration/coordination.

However, experience suggests that defining key tasks for individual jobs, and identifying their contribution to the overall purpose, can be difficult in health services. There are many jobs whose success is intrinsically linked to the efforts of teams and which are legitimately interchangeable within the group. In that case, it may be better to think in terms of team ownership of key tasks and joint contribution criteria.

Structuring appraisal to meet the demands of performance management

An appraisal system is essential to any manager wishing to define performance. Appraisal can be conceived as a six-step process, in which managers seek to guide appraisees through sets of questions which help focus the efforts of individuals on their effective contribution. The process is as follows, with the questions for the appraisees noted at each step:

Step 1: Clarify purpose of job

The first question to be settled is fundamental. Why does my job exist, in relation to clients whom my organization is serving?

Step 2: Define 'key tasks'

Having established the overall job purpose, the next step is to break it down into areas of significant activity, which reflect priorities for the reporting period. The key tasks are statements of contribution from the individual, in response to these questions:

1   In which areas do I have personal responsibility for achieving results?
2   In which areas may any failure on my part damage overall performance of the work unit?
3   What do I do of significance that neither my line manager nor my other work unit colleagues contribute?

If an up-to-date job description exists, it may provide a basis for identifying key tasks. On the other hand, analysis conducted at this stage may guide the revision of an existing job description.

Step 3: Decide required standards of performance for each key task

The appraisee poses this question for each key task identified in Step 2. How will I know when I am contributing to an adequate standard? Standards of performance identified beforehand are crucial in allowing the appraisee to judge progress towards effective contribution. It is at this step that qualitative as well as quantitative measures of contribution can be utilized.

Step 4: Developing an improvement plan with specified targets for the appraisee for the forthcoming review period

The manager and appraisee review all the key tasks and target areas for improvement – that is, actions to be taken to move their contribution towards the required standards of performance within the coming review period. The acronym SMART is useful in defining the nature of a target:

S = simple – clear, understandable
M = measurable – quantity, quality, money, time
A = agreed – between manager and appraisee
R = realistic – possible in terms of appraisee's capability and experience
T = timely – reflects current priorities and is assessable within the review period.

The types of question appraisees need to address are:

1 What are the significant contributions I have to make to close the gap between actual and desired performance, according to key success factors identified by the organization?
2 Are my standards of performance and respective targets achievable?
3 Are they compatible with those of other post-holders?
4 Do they represent an appropriate balance between my work and my personal development objectives?
5 Will they stimulate and motivate me, or exhaust and discourage me or others?
6 What data will I need in order to know whether I have met my targets? How will they be collected, analysed and made available to me?

Step 5: Initiate the period of the plan and monitor performance against targets

Regular monitoring and review are the only effective means for performance appraisal to become an integral part of the management process.

Step 6: The role of appraisal at the close of the plan period

The following questions are addressed by appraisees with the assistance of their appraisers.

1 How far have standards of performance been met in the key tasks of my job?
2 Did I achieve the targets according to the conditions set? If not, to what extent was I responsible for any shortfall?
3 How well did I utilize resources in achieving results?
4 What skills and competencies did I demonstrate in working towards target achievement?
5 Did I achieve any targets at the expense of other people/activities?

6 If factors outside my control constrained progress, how did I respond?
7 Was my overall performance in line with the plan, or did it exceed expectations/fail to meet expectations?

Levels of achievement of required standards of performance and targets are part of the context for determining the next year's work plan. They also stimulate discussion of the type and volume of future work demands on the appraisee, through two questions:

1 How much responsibility and new experience will I be able to take on?
2 Are there deficiencies in my knowledge, skill and experience that need to be addressed if I am to succeed with the next work plan?

✎ Activity 10.1

Considering your own performance in your own organization (and assuming you have had an appraisal):

1 Which targets for your performance, agreed at the last appraisal, have been:

(a) exceeded;   (b) met;   (c) not achieved?

2 What do you feel you have done particularly well *by your own standards* over the past 12 months?
3 What do you feel you have done least well *by your own standards* over the past 12 months?
4 To help improve your performance in the job still further, what additional steps could be taken by:

(a) you;   (b) your manager;   (c) others in the organization?

5 What changes, if any, in your responsibilities would you like to see in the near future?
6 What training and development steps could further your career development?

↻ Feedback

This activity should have given you a practical application of Step 6 above. In the next part of this chapter you will see how performance appraisal works in the practice of health services and how it can be linked with career management.

The purpose of formal appraisal

Formal appraisal arises from the need to collect and exchange information on employees' performance in a systematic manner. It enables managers to focus on the most salient features for improving performance. Most organizations undertake some form of appraisal, though not necessarily in the form presented above. A review of UK organizations by the Institute for Personnel Management (1992) suggested a range of key purposes associated with formal appraisal (Table 10.1).

Table 10.1 The uses of appraisal

Purpose	Percentage of organizations using formal appraisal for this purpose
To review past performance	98
To help improve current performance	97
To assess training and development needs	97
To set performance objectives	81
To assist career-planning decisions	75
To assess future potential/promotion	71
To assess salary increases	40

Source: Institute for Personnel Management (1992)

In large health care organizations, appraisal is usually by managers. Managers or senior staff members are the appraisers and staff are the appraisees, but other approaches do exist, including:

- *Upward assessment*, in which managers are appraised by their own staff; although still uncommon in health care organizations, this approach is being used in the private sector.
- *Peer group assessment*, which allows colleagues or team members to appraise an individual; used, for example, in academic institutions.
- Approaches that allow managers, peers and subordinates to participate as equals in appraisal, sometimes referred to as '*360 degree feedback*'.

Whilst these alternatives operate with principles different from the more usual top-down approach, some advantages and shortcomings may be common to all types of appraisal.

Introducing a performance appraisal system

To be effective, the objectives and principles of an appraisal system must be accepted throughout an organization, and its design and implementation need to be professional. For example, a study into a private hospital by Wilson and Cole (1990) attributed successful appraisal systems to their clarity of aims, careful design, and (crucially) keeping the staff involved throughout such that their own personal development needs were prioritized.

The appraisal interview

Activity 10.2

Imagine that you are to undertake *appraisal interviews* of all staff in a hospital. Outline what you think are the best ways in which the process should be conducted?

Feedback

The appraisal style should be open and positive, encouraging learning and change for the better. It assumes that any individual, with proper guidance and encouragement, can identify their own shortcomings and therefore has a better chance of being committed to putting them right, compared to individuals who are simply told that they are doing badly. The following guidelines assist the appraiser in guiding and encouraging appraisees.

1 Establish ownership of appraisal by encouraging appraisees to talk about their attitudes and feelings as well as their performance.

2 Further strengthen rapport by asking questions, like 'How do you think this could be improved?'; 'What about actions in this area?'; 'How would that affect the situation?'.

3 Give specific rather than general feedback and avoid valuation judgements so that appraisees do not react defensively.

4 Avoid emphasizing problems over which appraisees have no control.

5 Encourage appraisees to ask questions to elicit your response and feedback.

6 Present information so that appraisees can accept it without feeling devalued or blamed.

Any appraiser or supplier of feedback must be prepared to receive some views in return. There is more potential for trust if the appraiser is ready to receive feedback and to learn about the effect of his or her behaviour on others. This is important because performance improvement by the appraisee may require some change in supervision behaviour, which the appraisee must feel confident will occur. Thus the supervisor should be prepared to give something as well, rather than exclusively focusing on the appraisee.

Appraisal and career development

During appraisals appraisers can advise appraisees on career development opportunities and recommend promotion or sideways moves that are appropriate for both the organization and the individuals concerned. In addition, when career structures are changing because of the impact of technology, competitive pressure or the need for retrenchment, managers may also be required to inform employees of changes that affect their careers, such as restructuring job roles, and to encourage their adaptability to retain their interest and commitment. Appraisers are rarely able to avoid communicating such changes or probing employees on how they intend to respond to them. At the very least, managers can help employees prepare for change in relation to possible career moves.

Career management and development: a conceptual basis

Career choice within any organization is influenced by the type of organization it is and its values concerning the nature and duration of careers within the organization. The implication of this for career management is that there are limits to strategic choices that can be made. The most important choices (Armstrong, 1995) are:

1 Adopt career management systems that develop people for the longer term *or* be prepared to purchase skilled staff from the labour market when needed.
2 Invest in career development activities *or* leave career development entirely to individuals.
3 Encourage generalists who may be multi-skilled *or* ensure that appropriate specialists are in place.
4 Facilitate fast-track career development with specific needs in mind *or* provide broad career development to ensure a flexible response as different needs arise.
5 Remove managers who have reached their final career destination on the basis of current abilities *or* rehabilitate them, perhaps through lateral moves or special projects.

How such choices are made affects the nature of the interaction between appraisers and appraisees, and sets limits to the evolution of career opportunities for individuals. If a career system is in place, as for nurses or doctors in a hospital, then Edgar Schein's 'career path' is a useful concept for analysing how opportunities are taken up (Schein, 1977). He suggests a three-stage model of careers, which is developed below.

1 Entry point

Individuals enter the career on the basis of a specified standard at the recruitment stage, such as graduation from medical or nursing school.

2 Growing grades

These represent the lower rungs of career structures which entail the exercise of the specialist skills for which the staff member was recruited. Employees progress through the growing grades fairly automatically after recruitment, with an implicit guarantee of reaching the top of these grades unless performance falls well below expectation. For an employee not to reach the top of the growing grades usually reflects a recruitment mistake.

3 Significant job steps

These represent major promotions for individuals where they take on levels of responsibility, usually supervisory or managerial, for which they need to be carefully selected. There is an implication that staff will be developed to cope with the new types of demand on them. Appraisal generates key information on an individual's experience and achievement, and is used in selection for promotion and development.

Advocates of career paths maintain they are essential to career development as they provide the main source of information for employees to make choices about personal advancement. For the organization, they provide a way of ensuring that jobs relate to strategic goals by identifying the key attributes post-holders should possess and how those attributes should be developed.

Critics argue that structured career paths do not accommodate the dynamics of either organizational or individual change, and suggest two problems:

- Too much weight is given to how careers have evolved in the past – an organization's future work needs are likely to shift in response to a variety of environmental stimuli, thereby undermining the relevance of historical career tracks.
- A career progression pattern as currently reported may be misleading because it expresses an historic combination of individual qualifications and organizational needs that may now be redundant.

For example, doctors who have traditionally pursued a career in hospitals may find themselves confined to a career in primary care because of a downsizing of the hospital sector. In such circumstances, what employees perceive as career progression may not happen for them, with a negative impact on their expectations and motivation, and hence on organizational performance.

There is a danger then that appraisers and appraisees may rely too much on historical patterns of career progression when assessing prospects for appraisees. Also, the approach accentuates the idea that the natural route of development of abilities is towards supervision and management, rather than allowing for changes of working area or sideways transfers, which are more common today.

Issues in conducting appraisals in a performance management system

The advent of performance management systems, with their strategic approach to managing organizational and individual performance, places appraisal of performance in a central role in the management of human resources.

Activity 10.3

Thinking about the process of appraisal and specifically its potential as a tool for performance management:

1 what are the potential strengths of the approach?
2 what are its weaknesses?
3 to what extent would you agree with the statement that 'formal appraisal is an idea whose time has gone'?

Feedback

1 Potentially, appraisal of performance offers a great opportunity to motivate people and improve performance through objective setting and reviewing performance. The approach can be used as a tool for identifying and supporting staff training and development needs. Linking rewards to performance (such as in forms of performance-related pay) is more controversial but may provide specific incentives for tasks to be achieved.

2 The first problem is that appraisal often sets an overly demanding agenda such that seeking rewards for effort limits constructive discussions about development needs. Second, to impose performance management on traditionally managed public service organizations without adequate preparation is folly. Such organizations may lack an ongoing and open dialogue on what constitutes effective performance. Third, some areas of work in the health sector do not easily fit the methodology of performance management (giving health policy advice, for instance), but this is not necessarily recognized when systems are introduced. Fourth, it is equally fruitless to set sophisticated standards of job performance in organizations that lack adequate information systems to produce the necessary control data. And finally, individual target setting is nearly always poor in promoting teamwork.

3 The need for appraisal remains important as a performance management and development tool for staff.

The future for appraisal should move away from a monolithic, rigid system towards more flexible processes. A model put forward by Deming (1986) – 'managing for results' – stresses an appraisal system based on how results are achieved, rather than attributing results solely to the efforts and skills of individuals. Its key idea is the need to build trust between co-workers, which prevents planning and coordination being confused and possibly distorted, by behaviour induced by setting individual objectives. Table 10.2 demonstrates how Deming's approach to appraisal is geared towards assessing how individuals *work with others* to achieve results. The 'how' becomes much more significant than the 'what', with appraisal geared to teamwork, quality delivery systems for clients, managing work flows across traditional boundaries and engaging in dialogue that can generate new ideas for improving

Table 10.2 Reforming performance management towards meaningful measures of work outcomes

Measuring results		
targets imposed on individuals by managers and judged by them →	agreement of individual targets that relate to customer needs, jointly reviewed by manager and appraisee →	group judgement of the outcomes of efforts to improve key delivery systems for customers
Reviewing development needs		
managers' perceived view of training needs →	training related to work unit performance standards →	training related to level of individual capability and client feedback
Job contribution		
based on historic circumstances or whim →	conceived within a functional framework →	based on needs arising from systems of evaluation for measuring client satisfaction

Source: Adapted from Deming (1986)

service delivery. As appraisers, managers thus become increasingly concerned with measuring both individual *and* team contributions in the quest for effective service delivery.

Summary

In this chapter you have learnt about the use of performance management systems in health care organizations. Such systems begin with the identification of objectives that are then translated into required contributions of individual jobs or teams. You also saw that whilst appraisal can assist staff in their career development, there are also critical issues to be resolved in achieving positive impacts on staff attitudes and efforts through performance and appraisal.

References

Armstrong, M. (1995) *Personnel Management Practice*. London: Kogan Page.
Deming, W. E. (1986) *Out of the Crisis*. Cambridge, Massachusetts: MIT Institute for Advanced Engineering Study.
Humble, J. (1970) *Management by Objectives in Action*. Maidenhead: McGraw-Hill.
Institute for Personnel Management (1992) *Performance Management in the UK: An Analysis of the Issues*. London: IPM.
Reddin, W. (1971) *Managerial Effectiveness*. Maidenhead: McGraw-Hill.
Schein, E. H. (1977) *Career Dynamics: Matching Individual and Organizational Needs*. London: Addison-Wesley.

Managing interprofessional relationships

11

Overview

Managers in health care need to recognize that staff are often also members of a professional group. As well as behaving as individuals, they often behave as members of that group. In order to manage them, you will therefore need to know how these groups (and their members) are likely to behave in different circumstances. That is the ground you will cover in this chapter.

Learning objectives

After working through this chapter you will be able to:

- **understand why professional groups tend to work as enclaves;**
- **describe a number of reasons why different health care professions find it difficult to communicate with each other;**
- **consider ways of improving the communications between different health care professions.**

Key terms

Group think The way members of a group distort their thinking to become overly supportive of suggestions made within the group and dismissive of suggestions and challenges made from outside it.

Tribalism The tendency of members in a profession to engage in the phenomenon known as 'group think'.

Relationships between different health care professions

Although all health care professions share a concern for the well-being of the patient, there is often friction between members of different professions. Whilst some is due to the differences between individuals, that you have studied in previous chapters, much of it arises because of the way the professions view each other and that, in turn, arises out of the nature of the care they are providing.

Causes of friction between professions

As Iles (1997) describes, friction between the health care professions has resulted in part from the increased specialization of their roles and the growing *interdependencies* between them. Large, complex health care organizations have great numbers of interdependent professions and this can bring about problems of communication, a lack of shared understanding and fragmentation of responsibility.

Group think

Entering a health care profession may have been an ethical or moral decision based on the wish to care for others. However, despite the fact that most health care professionals are concerned with patient outcomes, it is often the case that their beliefs and values differ, leading to conflicting views.

First described by Janis (1971), 'group think' describes the tendency of members within the same cultural, political and/or professional groups to become overly supportive of suggestions made within their 'enclave' or 'clan' and dismissive of suggestions and challenges made from outside it. In health care organizations it is common to encounter such professional elites. You may recognize the principal characteristics (Iles, 1997, p. 20):

1 Group members are intensely loyal to the group and its policies, even if some of the consequences of the policies disturb the conscience of each member.
2 Members do not criticize the reasoning or the behaviour of fellow members. In Janis's words, the group is '*soft-headed*' because they have an unwavering belief in their own morality.
3 Members are also what Janis describes as '*hard-hearted*' when it comes to views of outsiders. They hold negative and prejudiced views against other groups and their leaders.
4 Individual members doubt and suppress their own reasoning when it conflicts with the reasoning of the group.
5 If a member *does* question the validity of arguments expressed, then the rest of the group will apply subtle coercive pressure for conformity.

Janis (1971) makes some recommendations about how managers can counteract group think. If you have problems with managing professional elites, Iles suggests posting these points on the wall of your office, or perhaps on your website:

1 Group leaders must validate the importance of critical evaluation of all views.
2 Leaders should require each member to discuss group deliberations with associates in other groups.
3 The group should invite external consultants to challenge the views of members.
4 Members should be encouraged to play devil's advocate.
5 Whenever a group's deliberations involve relations with a rival organization, they should devote time to finding out as much as possible about their rivals and consider alternative ways of interpreting what the group perceives to be hostile action.

Activity 11.1

1 Call to mind a group of which you are a member and with which you identify closely. It could be your professional group or a team you belong to socially. Consider the features of group think listed above. Do they apply to your group? If they do, write down an example of each feature.

2 Consider which of Janis's five suggestions for preventing group think may be possible in your team.

3 How do you feel about the prospect of challenging the group's thinking in these ways? Are you reluctant to do so? Is the comfort of the group too important to you?

4 Make a list of some groups you work with who engage in group think, noting an example of the ideas they are 'soft-headed' about and the people or groups about whom they are 'hard-hearted'.

Feedback

If you answered 'yes' to Question 1 then you have a personal example of how the self-censorship that Janis describes works. Now that you are aware of the phenomenon of group think, you will be able to choose not to engage in it yourself. Sometimes your membership of a group will feel too important to you and you will not want to risk the displeasure of the other members by challenging their soft-headedness or their hard-heartedness. This is a moral decision for you and no one else can make it for you; now you have the awareness to know that you have a choice and that there will be consequences of that choice. You are also aware of the group think engaged in by other groups. If their soft-headedness or hard-heartedness is inhibiting good patient care then you can refer back to Janis's five ideas on how to challenge their perceptions.

Causes of tribalism

Iles (1997) outlines four further causes of 'tribal' behaviour in professionals.

The hierarchy of clinical descriptions

The nature of medical descriptions (Blois, 1984) reveals that there is a hierarchy in the way conditions are described. Hence, a child may say 'my mother is very tired and weak', whilst the doctor may have identified a specific type of cancer. Blois categorized this type of difference as follows:

Level +2	patient's community
Level +1	patient's family
Level 0	patient as a whole
Level −1	major body part (e.g. chest)
Level −2	physiological system (e.g. respiratory system)
Level −3	system part or organ (e.g. lung)
Level −4	organ part or tissue (e.g. myocardium)

Level −5   cell (e.g. lymphocyte, fibroblast)
Level −6   cell part (e.g. membrane, nucleus)
Level −7   macromolecule (e.g. enzyme, protein)
Level −8   micromolecule (e.g. glucose, ascorbic acid)
Level −9   atoms or ions (e.g. sodium ion)

There are three key features that need to be understood about this hierarchy. First, there is a 'health care pathway' in which you can track experiences between the various levels, from the widest health of a society to the smallest part of the human anatomy. Second, each level has its own 'language', often from general terms with wide meaning to complicated terminology with very specific meanings. Third, professionals tend to have expertise at the different layers, rather than between them.

The implication of the hierarchy is that managers of health care organizations need to be concerned with each level – not just illness (minus numbers) but also patient and society well-being (positive numbers). Furthermore, managers need to overcome communication difficulties between the layers as a result of language and group think, and understand the value of each layer in the process of care (Iles, 1997).

The spectrum of the views of disease

In the same way that clinical hierarchies result in group think, so too is the contrast between those that have a traditional biomedical view of treating illness with the more holistic or social view of treating the person. The former is concerned with the specifics of treating a disease as if it were in isolation of the patient, the second favours patient well-being. The tension between the medical and the social model of care has often been documented, for example in the care management of older people with complex chronic conditions.

The degree of structure in a clinical problem

A third key cause of tribalism is the breadth of knowledge required of a health care professional during a patient encounter. Thus, in first contact care with a generalist where the patient's concerns could be anything or nothing, the widest range of options must first be considered. As more knowledge is known about a patient's condition, so the more narrow and specialist the field of enquiry becomes. In health care, generalists are often less valued or trusted by specialists in the care of a patient since they have less knowledge of specific conditions. However, generalists are essential in the care pathway. Thus, professionals need to recognize the value of different roles and skills in providing care, rather than greater or less skill in the treatment process.

Philosophical stances

The philosophical stance of a profession can often be very different to your own. Where individuals are unaware of other beliefs or fundamentally disagree with another's point of view, communication between them is virtually impossible since it invokes an emotional response as much as a logical one. For both parties to make progress, each must be willing to look at their own underlying beliefs to question and discuss them.

Communication difficulties

Many of the tensions between professions, or between branches of the same profession, arise out of the difference in their tasks. The following case study describes a real incident which took place in England in 1992 (Anon, 1992). The incident is presented by one of the people involved but gives information about, and letters from, the other party. There may not be direct parallels in your health care system, so use the case as an opportunity to diagnose some of the issues you have read about, and to consider how you may use them.

The road to hell

In January 1991 Mr George Harris was taken ill and admitted to his local hospital, Shire District Hospital. It had no empty beds for male patients, so he was sent to St Emily's Hospital, five miles away. While he was in hospital his wife was also taken ill and was admitted to Shire District Hospital.

After several days Mr Harris, an elderly, partially sighted non-insulin dependent diabetic, came home, but within four or five hours it became clear to me, his general practitioner, that he was still unwell. The following is an abridged version of the correspondence (names and places have been changed) which occurred after I failed to gain his admission to the district hospital so that he had to be sent back to St Emily's Hospital where he died some two weeks later.

There is no right and wrong here; there are different views. But the correspondence also shows an inability on the part of some doctors to move out of their way of thinking and see another perspective. The idea of printing the letters is to provoke discussion about priorities and values in medicine, so that general practitioners and hospital doctors can work out an appropriate and responsive way of working.

Extract of letter from admitting general practitioner to consultant (Dr Brown) at Shire District Hospital who had refused to admit Mr Harris (January 1991):

'I am writing to you to register my protest over the events which occurred last Friday night.

'I felt that [Mr Harris's] condition merited [re]admission, and in view of the fact that his wife is in your hospital it seemed to me that it would be appropriate to admit him [there].

'According to your senior house officer you [had] two available male medical beds but both he and you refused to admit this patient and advised me to send him back to St Emily's Hospital. Mr and Mrs Harris are a very frail elderly couple and it is quite likely that any illness may be their last.

'Medical tradition urges us to "cure when possible, comfort frequently and care always"; it strikes me that to force a couple unnecessarily into separate hospitals is cruel. Unfortunately it reinforces my impression that certain aspects of hospital medicine are more concerned with syndromes and illnesses and less with patients and their needs as people.

'It is also worth mentioning that the Harris' relatives are [now] obliged to commute five miles twice daily in two different directions, which is unreasonable.

'My purpose in writing is to emphasise the human side of illness; it is vital that all doctors retain an awareness of the vulnerability of their patients and not lose touch with their "non-medical" needs. I fear that this has happened here, and I hope it does not happen again.'

Extract of letter from Dr Brown to general practitioner (this letter was sent on the same day as the first one, and they crossed in the post);

'I understand from my SHO (Dr Smythe) that you are making a complaint to the unit general manager as to my decision over the weekend and you also made comments as to this hospital's attitude towards patient care. These witnessed comments are documented and I will welcome your complaint so that it may be subject to full formal assessment by your and my peers and the appropriate remedial action taken if unprofessional behaviour is uncovered.'

Extract of letter from chairman of Shire District Hospital medical division to the general practitioner (February 1991):

'The medical division considered your letter of complaint concerning Mr George Harris. Medical division was extremely concerned about several features of your letter.

'(1) You seem to be unaware of the critical nature of our bed state recently. Several times patients with severe medical problems have had to be sent to St Emily's Hospital because there have been no beds available.

'This is due to a combination of bad weather and the relative underprovision of medical beds. The latter factor has been with us for a long time and is only manageable if all parties concerned exert the maximum goodwill and common sense in using scarce resources.

'In favour of Mr Harris's admission to Shire Hospital rather than St Emily's was the fact that his wife was a patient [here].

'Against admission of Mr Harris to Shire District was the fact that all [his] notes, x rays, and blood tests would be available at St Emily's, and that he would be known to the medical team there.

'Also against admitting the patient to Shire District Hospital was the fact that there were only two available male medical beds, and this at the start of a weekend, when admissions are often numerous and discharges are less common.

'A balanced decision had to be taken and Dr Smythe and Dr Brown felt that Mr Harris should be readmitted to St Emily's Hospital.

'Medical division felt that the correct decision had been made, as did Dr Raleigh, who was Mr Harris's consultant at St Emily's.

'However, they were extremely concerned that your disagreement led you to state that the decision was "inhumane and cruel" and to say that you feel that "certain aspects of hospital medicine are more concerned with syndromes and illnesses and less with patients and their needs as people."

'Medical division was shocked and saddened that you should take this view of the care provided at your local hospital by your medical colleagues and We are rather indignant about the fact that you should write to Dr Brown in this way, with a copy to the unit general manager and district general manager, when a personal discussion might have been more appropriate. This would have given you the opportunity to improve any defects you perceive in the system, and allow mutual education about the situation in which general practitioners find themselves working.

'(2) I [will] contact the secretary of the local medical committee to find out whether the local general practitioners as a body would share your views, in which case it may be relevant to arrange a meeting between hospital staff and GPs.

'(3) We have discussed these events with Dr Smythe, the on call SHO. He quite correctly discussed the matter of Mr Harris's admission with Dr Brown at the time of the request.

'We are told that . . . you wished to prolong the discussion with Dr Smythe and when he said that he would have to terminate the discussion in order to look after a critically ill patient in diabetic coma, you accused him of trying to put the "phone down on you" and informed him that you were going to complain formally to Dr Brown and the unit general manager.

'You also commented that you hoped that Dr Smythe was not one of the hospital's GP trainees. As you are now aware, Dr Smythe has already completed a general practitioner vocational training scheme and is a member of the Royal College of General Practitioners, although he has decided that his future lies in hospital medicine.

'Nevertheless, if Dr Smythe had been one of the hospital's GP trainees, medical division feel that he may have felt threatened by your attitude and this is something which we totally deplore.

'(4) Medical division feels that an apology is due to Dr Brown for the offensive suggestion that his team were "inhumane and cruel." '

Extract of letter from the general practitioner to the chairman of the medical division (February 1991):

'I am writing in response to your letter, which I found rather depressing. It is important that the issue is clarified, so that such a problem will not occur again.

'Firstly, it is not and never has been my habit to make "formal complaints" about any difficulties with the health service. Like you, I am much happier with informal discussions, which avoid confrontations of this sort.

'The first time that the phrase occurred was in the letter which Dr Brown sent to me in January. I am enclosing a copy of this letter [above], and ask you to consider it in the light of the sentence in your letter which reads: "We are rather indignant about the fact that you should write to Dr Brown in this way . . . when a personal discussion might have been more appropriate."

'My wish was merely to "protest over the events which took place"; I sent a copy to the district general manager because he has previously encouraged me to let him know if I ever encountered problems with any aspect of Shire's delivery of health care.

'From the points of view of myself, both my patients, and their relatives, there was a problem, hence my letter.

'Secondly, I am grateful that the medical division has given the problem so much thought. If item 2 in your letter really leads to better liaison between the hospital and the primary care physicians, then some good will have come from this whole sad saga . . .'

Activity 11.2

1   Who held the clinical responsibility for Mr Harris?
2   Why did the telephone conversation become so acrimonious so quickly?
3   What were the concerns of the GP?
4   How were they addressed by the hospital doctor?
5   What were the concerns of the hospital doctor?
6   How were they addressed by the GP?

Feedback

1 The case is an example of the responsibility for care being shared and of problems arising at the boundary between two groups within one profession (medicine).

2 The telephone conversation became acrimonious very quickly which suggests that both parties *expected* the other to behave unreasonably; in other words, each held a negative stereotyped view of the other prior to the conversation. This may be a symptom of group think occurring in both general practitioners and hospital doctors.

3–6 The GP is concerned about level 0 and level +1 in the hierarchy of clinical descriptions (the patient and family). The hospital doctor is thinking of how best to deal with level −8. Each is arguing for the best outcome for the level they are considering but they are not addressing the concerns of the other. Similarly, the GP has greater knowledge of this patient and the family, and the hospital has greater expertise in the treatment of this clinical condition. They are operating at different points on the spectrum of disease, without acknowledging it. The hospital doctor is also concerned with other potential patients who may need the bed. This concern is not addressed by the GP. Their philosophical stances appear to be similar so that is not a cause of the communication difficulties here.

Activity 11.3

Put yourself in the position of the GP. Imagine how you would be feeling and what you would be thinking.

1   How would you prepare for making the initial telephone call?
2   What would you say?
3   How would you respond if the reaction to your request was 'We cannot spare any beds here, send him to St Emily's'?

Feedback

Compare your answers with those that follow and use any differences as a basis for reflecting on how you would choose to approach a situation in which you disagreed with another professional (or a patient or their family) about the best course of action.

1 Before making the telephone call you, the GP, must decide that your *care* for your patient will require you to undertake 'acts of work, and acts of courage'. In this case the *work* will include:

- considering carefully the situation of your patient;
- identifying the care options available;
- planning thoroughly the conversations you must have with other care providers (including the hospital);
- accepting responsibility for the nature of the relationship with other care providers;
- mastering your feelings of irritation or anger. It will help you to do this if, when you experience anger or irritation, you try to identify the fear that lies at the root of it. Is your fear warranted? What can you do to avoid the consequences you fear? When you think of an answer to the last question then do that rather than giving in to anger or irritation.

The *courage* may be needed:

- to make the telephone call to someone you believe may be argumentative or obstructive;
- to break bad news to the family;
- to encourage the family to work constructively with whatever option the other care providers allow.

2 When you make the telephone call, you must have a strategy ready for dealing with whichever conflict mode you diagnose the hospital doctor to be in. You may assume that they will have a shortage of beds and be under pressure from senior staff not to accommodate your wishes. They are likely to be in competitive (a win–lose) mode. You need them to move to collaborative mode and can only achieve that by persuading them of the problem as you perceive it. Thus, instead of starting the conversation with your preferred solution ('I want you to admit this patient'), you are more likely to be successful if you describe your problem ('I have a patient who . . .'). You are unlikely to have the psychological equilibrium to do this if the patient's family are in the room. If you feel that the other doctor is not responding to your problem you can try using the 'broken record' technique of repeating it, calmly, until he or she acknowledges that there is indeed a problem to be solved.

3 If you meet a 'brick wall' of 'no, I cannot admit your patient', then you need to try and establish exactly what the hospital doctor's problems are. When both sets of problems are out in the open you have all the information you need to try and design a solution, jointly, which meets both your needs. It may not be your preferred option. It may, for example, mean transferring your patient's wife to St Emily's hospital, but you will be no worse off than if you choose to become angry. And you will have established a more constructive relationship which may yield results in the future.

Summary

You have learnt how professions often exhibit a syndrome of faulty perceptions and suboptimal reasoning which is called group think. When professions operate at different levels in the hierarchy of clinical descriptions, they are bound to find communication difficult, they will require different kinds of evidence on which to base their decisions, and they will need help to consider all the relevant factors in a decision. Not all health care professionals are explicit about how they define health and very many have never attempted to define care. Doing so enables professionals to prepare for and conduct negotiations with other professionals in a constructive way. Entering into any negotiation involves making choices about how to behave.

References

Anon (1992) The road to hell, *British Medical Journal*, 304 (6827): 628–9.

Blois, M. (1984) *Information and Medicine: The Nature of Medical Descriptions*. Stanford: University of California Press.

Iles, V. (1997) *Really Managing Health Care*. Buckingham: Open University Press.

Janis, I. (1971) Group-think, *Psychology Today*, reprinted in J. Hackman, E. Lawler and L. Porter (eds) (1983) *Perspectives on Behaviour in Organizations*. New York: McGraw-Hill, pp. 378–84.

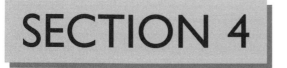

SECTION 4

Managing results

12 | **Evaluating performance**

Overview

In this and the next two chapters you will learn about measuring the performance of health services and how such information can be used to manage and improve the quality of care. In this chapter you will be introduced to three measures: productivity, capacity and speed of delivery.

Learning objectives

After you have worked through this chapter you will be able to:

- **describe the need for performance measurement;**
- **define measures of productivity, capacity, capacity utilization and speed of delivery;**
- **consider the measures that are most appropriate for any given service;**
- **describe how to compare the performance of organizations (benchmarking) and its uses.**

Key terms

Benchmarking The process of comparing performance against that of the leaders in a particular industry or against targets.

Capacity A measure of the maximum possible output performance that an organizational unit can achieve over a given time period.

Capacity utilization A measure of the extent to which the potential maximum capacity of an organization is being used.

Productivity A measure of how efficiently inputs are converted into outputs.

The need for measuring and evaluating performance

Performance evaluation of a health care system or organization is needed if managers are to understand how best to develop and control what is occurring within it. Performance evaluation is the way most managers can formally assess whether their organization is meeting the needs of its clients (users or patients). If you do not measure how well an individual, a team or an organization is performing, you cannot know how well they are performing and so you cannot make changes, provide guidance and support, which will improve their performance to the level needed to improve organizational outcomes.

Types of performance measure

The way you measure *performance* will differ according to the kind of job, service or organization you are looking at. However, there are some common types of performance measure.

Productivity

One of the most commonly used measures is that of *productivity*, which measures how efficiently you convert inputs into outputs. For example, in a company manufacturing shoes the outputs would be the total number of shoes produced in a given period. The inputs would include staff, materials, equipment and rent for the premises. There are three different kinds of productivity measure:

1 A *partial measure* would include just one or two of the inputs, for example: labour productivity = outputs / staff costs or staff hours.
2 A *multi-factor measure* includes several inputs, for example: outputs / staff materials and equipment.
3 A *total measure* includes all the inputs.

Partial measures are most often used because it is usually one variable that is the most critical. This variable differs from industry to industry. For example, for a restaurant it may be meals per staff hour; in a shop it would be turnover (sales) per square metre; on a farm it may be tons of wheat per hectare.

On its own, a productivity measure of this kind would tell you very little. When you compare it with past performance then you can tell whether productivity is increasing, decreasing or remaining constant. If you compare it with another company or team, then you can see if you are doing better than, worse than or the same as other people.

Capacity and capacity utilization

It is useful to know the *capacity* of a team, service or centre in terms of the output they can achieve. Again the measure will differ with the industry. In a restaurant it could be customers; in a factory making cars it would be cars per week; in a hospital it could be the number of in-patients per night; for a home nursing service it may the number of appointments per week.

Often capacity is measured at two levels: optimal capacity (the capacity a unit was designed to turn out) and maximum capacity (what it can turn out for short periods if it has to, but with greater wear and tear costs).

Once you have ascertained the capacity you can measure *capacity utilization*. Capacity utilization is the relationship between the optimal capacity an organizational unit can achieve in comparison to the actual output. Again, this is most useful when compared with past performance or with the performance of another team or organization; and again a poor result should prompt you to ask questions of the team involved rather than take immediate action. Of course, persistent inability to reach satisfactory capacity utilization would mean that you had resources being wasted by not being used.

Speed of delivery

The length of time between receiving an order and delivering the goods or services is a measure that is very important to the customer. In health care this is manifest in waiting times for appointments. Although useful in its own right, the waiting time is either acceptable or it is unacceptable, in which case some remedial action must be taken – it is again most useful when compared with past performance or with other organizations. It is this comparison that allows you to investigate the situation, to evaluate changes that have been made and to devise new ways of tackling the problem.

Benchmarking

Benchmarking is the process of comparing performance against that of the leaders in your industry. You look not only at performance measures but at how this leading organization or team achieves these performance levels. When you have identified their good practices you might investigate how to implement them in your own organization or team.

Performance measures in your organization

Now that you have read about how to measure performance, here is an opportunity for you to measure your own.

✎ Activity 12.1

1 Does anyone measure your productivity? If yes, what outputs do they measure?
2 Do you think this is the most appropriate measure of productivity? If no, what would be the most appropriate measure?
3 If your productivity is measured, has it increased, decreased or remained the same over the past year?

  If increased, what reasons could there be for your performance increasing?
  If decreased, what reasons could there be for your performance decreasing?

4 If your chief executive wanted a total measure of the productivity of your team or department, what would you include in the inputs? (Suggestions: staff costs, material and equipment costs, costs of premises, cost of manager.)
5 What is your optimal capacity? (The output you can achieve on a regular basis if fully occupied.)

6 What is your maximum capacity? (The output you can achieve if working very hard.)
7 How long could you work at maximum capacity before needing some time off to recuperate?
8 What is your capacity utilization?

   Actual outputs / optimal outputs

9 What reasons could there be for your capacity utilization increasing?
10 Is there a waiting list for your services?

   If so, what is your waiting time (the length of time people have to wait for your service)? If you have no waiting list this will be zero.

11 If you were to benchmark your department or team, what measure of performance would you employ?
12 Which department or team would you choose to compare your performance with? (Remember, this should be a leading team from whom you might be able to learn a lot.)

↻ Feedback

These questions were designed to allow you to focus on measures of your own organization's performance, so there are clearly no right or wrong answers.

A word about benchmarking – you may find that the productivity, capacity utilization or speed of delivery measure of the team you choose is no better than yours, yet you have considered them to be an excellent team, better (even) than you. So there are some important measures that you have not yet considered: measures of quality. That is the subject of the next chapter.

Summary

Performance must be measured if it is to be managed. It can be measured in a number of different ways the main measures being productivity (partial, multi-factor or total), capacity, capacity utilization and speed of delivery. There are also measures of quality and these are considered in the next chapter. To be most useful, measures need to be compared either to past performance or the performance of a competitor or other team/organization. If the measurement yields unsatisfactory results (productivity is decreasing, for example) then the next step is to ask questions of the individual or team concerned to find out why.

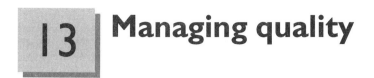

13 Managing quality

Overview

In this chapter you will learn about managing the quality of services. However, there are difficulties in doing this given the complexity of health care. To improve quality, measurement is essential but it is not enough. The work of some of the quality experts in manufacturing industries can provide useful lessons.

Learning objectives

After you have worked through this you will be able to:

- **define quality of care;**
- **describe the principles of total quality management;**
- **discuss the problems associated with measuring quality in health care;**
- **describe some quality measures;**
- **discuss the role of the manager in influencing the quality of health care.**

Key terms

Quality Features or characteristics of a product or service that demonstrate 'fitness for purpose' relating to their ability to meet stated needs.

Quality chain The chain of suppliers and customers of health services. The integrity of the chain is important for ensuring service quality is upheld.

Total quality management (continuous quality improvement) An approach to quality improvement that involves the commitment of all members of an organization to meeting the needs of its external and internal customers.

Why is quality important?

In both the private and the public sector, measuring and managing quality is essential for the following reasons:

1. You cannot claim to offer a high-quality product or service unless you measure its quality. You may feel you are doing a good job, but you cannot know unless you measure it in some way.
2. Measurement is not enough. It is the intention to change things for the better that leads to increased quality. People must *want* to increase the quality of what

they are doing if this is to happen. Their desire to work better must be informed by measurement of how well they are doing. Their desire to work better must be translated into action through systems set up to support them in doing so.

3 Quality must be built in. If quality is not built into products and services whilst they are being made, it cannot be added on later.

4 There must be commitment to quality from the most influential people in the organization. In health care organizations the most influential people may be key clinicians. If top people expect imperfection, then they get it. If they expect good performance, then their staff will develop the same expectations and meet them.

What does quality mean?

Quality is often defined as *fitness for purpose* (Juran, 1964). For example, if you want a car that is economical in the use of petrol, then a large high-performance model might be termed lower quality. However, to others the style, design, speed and comfort of the high-performance car might be seen as higher quality. It is because the purpose of a product or service is defined by the person receiving it that quality must be expressed in terms of both fitness for purpose and in terms of *meeting the needs of customers*.

Maxwell (1984) identified six dimensions of quality:

1 access to services
2 relevance to need (for the whole population)
3 effectiveness (for individual patients)
4 equity (fairness)
5 social acceptability
6 efficiency and economy

Activity 13.1

Describe how Maxwell's six dimensions of quality could be applied to your service or to a patient care service with which you are familiar.

Feedback

1 You may consider the accessibility of a service in a number of ways. For example, you may check on people's physical access:

- can people in wheelchairs reach you?
- how close are you to public transport?

Or you may consider any language barriers or financial barriers that reduce people's access.

2 To establish relevance to needs you would have to measure the needs of the population (which you learnt about in Chapters 7 to 11).

3 The effectiveness of care is the province of clinical audit. This can be undertaken in a number of different ways.

4 If receiving care is determined by factors other than their clinical, social and psychological needs, then your service may be inequitable. To measure this you would need to collect data about sex, age, race and so on, and analyse the care provided to see if there is a correlation between care options offered and particular groups.

5 Social acceptability can be ascertained by patient satisfaction surveys and reviewing patient complaints.

6 You studied some efficiency measures in the last chapter: for example, productivity and capacity utilization.

Whatever the list of factors, health care quality is primarily a measure of Juran's idea of 'fitness for purpose'. Thinking in these terms allows managers to set acceptable standards of care and assess performance against them.

Total quality management (TQM)

Total quality management (or continuous quality improvement) seeks to create a culture whereby all employees are continually examining and improving the organization of their work with a view to satisfying customer requirements. As the name implies, TQM focuses on quality as a key to organizational and managerial excellence. Joiner and Scholtes (1985) identified three key components:

1 the customer as the defining factor in determining quality;
2 teamwork as a means of unifying goals;
3 a scientific approach to decision-making based on data collection and analysis.

This 'Joiner Triangle' (Figure 13.1) is underpinned by a belief that organizational

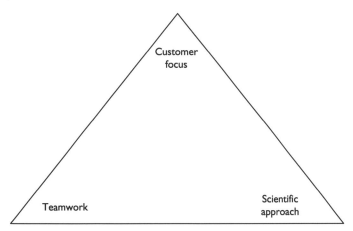

Figure 13.1 The 'Joiner Triangle' of total quality management
Source: Adapted from Joiner and Scholtes (1985)

defects are caused primarily by system failures rather than by the actions of individuals. Therefore, if you want to improve the quality of services you have to look at ways of improving systems and not just exhorting individuals to work harder or better. If something goes wrong, and a client suffers as a result, then any investigation should concentrate first on systems.

Customer focus

One of the main aims of TQM is customer satisfaction. In this sense, customers are not only patients but also clinical and non-clinical colleagues. If you meet their needs well then you are building quality in to the service offered by the organization as a whole. If you treat colleagues badly, then even if you personally meet the needs of your patients, you have not helped your colleagues to meet the needs of theirs and thus you have reduced quality where you could have improved it.

Activity 13.2

A hospital ward is not properly cleaned and several patients suffer from an illness as a result. You give a severe reprimand to the cleaning staff but you are told later that this may not have been the most productive way forward. Why were you given this advice and what alternative strategies do you think were available?

Feedback

There is a long supply chain to be considered here of which the cleaning staff are but one element. Hence the chain may involve: cleaners, cleaning supervisors, medical and nursing staff, maintenance staff, recruitment and training, pay scales, and the purchasing function right back to the suppliers of the cleaning material themselves, or even the beds and the layout of the wards themselves. The whole supply chain needs to be examined to discover the integrity and nature of the chain, not just the cleaning service itself. Keyser (1989) suggests you need to ask three key questions:

1 What do you need from me?

2 What do you do with what I give you?

3 Are there any gaps between what I give you and what you need?

This enables a better understanding of the apparently simple system of ward cleanliness and the points at which the system needs to be improved.

Teamwork

TQM seeks to create a climate or culture of teamwork where everyone is continuously striving to improve the quality of their work. This means getting everyone to work as part of a problem-solving team and to change management practices as a result. Brainstorming new ideas and examining feasible solutions is a natural remedy but the process of managing change in teams needs to be more structured – for example, in the use of force-field analysis and other approaches seeking to determine the forces and pressures in favour and against a potential change and its likely subsequent impact on the organization. Such processes will be reviewed in more detail in Chapters 15 to 17.

Scientific approach

A final key element to TQM is that quality should be scientifically designed into the systems which produce a service. Hence, if quality is built into every stage in the process of service development, then the final product – the service received by the patient – will be high quality. The typical scientific approach employs the plan-do-study-act (PDSA) cycle originally put forward by Deming (1982) (Figure 13.2).

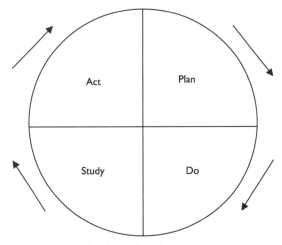

Figure 13.2 The Deming cycle (plan-do-study-act)

Source: Adapted from Deming (1982)

The four steps in the PDSA cycle are:

1 *Plan* the approach to a quality problem ensuring that all stakeholders are identified including all customers (patients) and all internal personnel involved in the service being delivered.
2 *Do* the experiment, or change, and collect data on the result.
3 *Study* the results, on a group basis, and examine whether the changes are working and are justified, and any delays that are present.
4 *Act* to incorporate the new methods (if they work) or revise them if they do not.

The quality chain

Every organizational system consists of a chain of suppliers and customers – what Morgan (1994) describes as a *quality chain*. This chain may be broken at any point where it is weak – for example, where one person or one piece of equipment does not meet the required standards. Failure to meet requirements leads to knock-on (or knock-back) effects, creating problems elsewhere. Failures in the chain often manifest themselves in poor services to customers, such as the delivery of faulty goods or delays in treatment. However, if the chain is managed so that no weaknesses exist, everyone in the chain benefits and maximum quality can be achieved.

The quality chain idea has been taken up by most organizations that have developed TQM programmes. The health of the quality chain can be examined in four discrete stages:

1 *Inspection*. Usually an after-the-fact screening process to assess the quality and conformity of services or products produced.
2 *Quality control*. Monitoring the process of service delivery at each stage in the chain in order to eliminate the causes of unsatisfactory performance.
3 *Quality assurance*. Assessment of the system's quality and the steps taken to improve quality.
4 *Total quality management*. The application of quality management principles at every level of the organization. This necessitates a change in behaviour amongst staff to commit to the quality management agenda.

Stages of quality management

TQM requires a significant degree of change management within a health care organization since it implies the development and acceptance of a quality management agenda throughout the organization which may be populated by those with different professional values, interdependencies and levels of clinical freedom. TQM is as much a tool to develop change management in an organization as to ensure that service quality is achieved. In developing TQM, Crosby (1979) identified five stages through which organizations generally pass. These five stages, from the least to the most desirable, are as follows:

1 *Uncertainty*. Characterized by management having no knowledge of quality as a positive management tool. As a result, problems are addressed on an *ad hoc* basis as and when they arise.
2 *Awakening*. Management begins to recognize that quality management is useful but is still reluctant and unwilling to commit resources to it. However, there is a realization that quality management can help.
3 *Enlightenment*. Management decides to implement TQM as it becomes committed to quality.
4 *Wisdom*. Managers and the whole organization reach a stage at which changes can be made as they identify problems in the quality chain. Employees and customers begin to actively participate in the quality improvement process.
5 *Certainty*. Management and the organization reach agreement on changes to be made. A preventive system is developed and quality improvement becomes accepted as standard practice.

Can you identify where your organization, or one you know well, sits along this five-stage model?

It has been argued that most public sector health care organizations remain in the awakening phase – that is, recognizing the value of TQM but continuing to fight problems on an *ad hoc* basis. Key reasons cited for this often include a lack of time and resources, and the reluctance to change within traditional professional practices.

Implementing TQM

There is no single approach to TQM that is 'right' for all health care organizations (Morgan, 1994). However, it is recognized that several elements need to be in place to help such organizations move in the direction of improving quality of care on a systematic basis. These include the availability of training, the development of teamwork, the development of a structure to support quality improvement, and a set of common measurable targets through which to assess change.

✎ Activity 13.3

Imagine you are the chief executive of your organization. Describe how you would influence the quality of clinical care by writing down a few words or phrases from the concepts you have studied in this chapter which come to mind in response to the following questions.

1 How would you persuade clinicians that measurement of the quality of their care is essential?
2 How would you encourage clinicians to want to improve their services?
3 How would you ensure that quality is built into all stages of services provision?
4 List the most influential people in the organization. How would you enthuse them with a commitment to quality?
5 How would you foster a shared belief that systems fail, not people?

↺ Feedback

Phrases you could have written down in response to these questions include the following.

1 Problem selling; robust relationships; expecting their best; opportunities for bench-marking; using statistics to ask questions.

2 Expecting their best; putting people back in touch with the personal vision; robust relationships; your commitment to quality; use of statistics to ask questions.

3 Empowerment: let the people closest to the patient design the systems.

4 You may have included managers and clinicians on your list, suggesting they might

be enthused by your own commitment to quality; robust relationships; challenge and support, work and courage.

5 Investigating system faults whenever there appears to be a people problem.

There are many more possibilities but the flavour is clear – the behaviour of a manager is more important than their ability to analyse statistics.

Summary

You have learned that the measurement of quality is essential but that measurement in itself is not enough – the intention to improve quality is also necessary. Quality can be defined as a service that is 'fit for purpose' and which meets the needs of the customer. TQM is an approach which stresses the importance of both internal customers as well as external ones. It also emphasizes that it is systems that fail, not people. However, finding measures of quality in health care is difficult because the services are complex. Managers must work through robust relationships across the quality chain to best influence the quality of clinical care.

References

Crosby, P. (1979) *Quality is Free*. New York: McGraw-Hill.

Deming, W. (1982) *Out of Crisis*. Massachusetts Institute of Technology, Boston.

Joiner, B. and Scholtes, P. (1985) *Total Quality Leadership vs Management by Control*. Joiner and Associates.

Juran, J. (1964) *Managerial Breakthrough*. New York: McGraw-Hill.

Keyser, W. (1989) Health care: is total quality relevant?, *Total Quality Management*, February: 20–32.

Maxwell, R. (1984) Quality assessment in health, *British Medical Journal*, 288(6428): 1470–2.

Morgan, P. (1994) Total quality management, in E. Monica (ed.) *Management in Health Care. A Theoretical and Experiential Approach*. Basingstoke: Palgrave MacMillan.

Further reading

Davies, H., Malek, M., Neilson, A. and Tavakoli, M. (eds) (1999) *Managing Quality: Strategic Issues in Health Care Management*. Aldershot: Ashgate.

Katz, J. and Green, E. (1996) *Managing Quality: Guide to Improving Performance in Health Care*, 2nd edn. London: Mosby.

14 Performance-related pay

Overview

In the last two chapters, managing efficiency and quality were presented as key approaches for managing results at an organizational level. In this chapter you will look specifically at using pay as an incentive for individuals or health care teams to improve organizational performance. However, as you will see, performance-related pay (PRP) is associated with pitfalls and problems of implementation in the health sector and is a blunt tool when confronted with the complex motivations of public sector employees. These issues will be discussed taking nursing as an example.

Learning objectives

After working through this chapter you will be able to:

- outline the features of a performance-related pay system;
- describe the problems of applying PRP to individual members of health care teams;
- conceptualize the interrelationship between work motivation and pay, and outline potential effects of PRP in health care organizations.

Key terms

Crowding-in A situation in which motivations of individuals to perform activities are increased by financial rewards.

Crowding-out A situation in which the professional or altruistic behaviours of individuals are adversely affected by direct remuneration for the task.

Expectancy theory A theory suggesting that the level of performance is directly related to the level of individual reward.

Instrumental work motivation A situation in which workers value work principally for the material rewards it provides.

Intrinsic work motivation A situation in which work is valued for itself rather than for its material rewards.

Performance-related pay A system that provides financial incentives to individuals and/or groups to work more effectively to meet measurable goals.

What is performance-related pay?

Performance-related pay can be seen as one approach to using pay to provide an *incentive* to individuals to work more effectively to meet organizational goals, both in terms of quality and efficiency. Armstrong and Murlis (1994) use it to refer to schemes that 'base additional financial rewards on ratings of performance, contribution and competence'. PRP, they say, has now 'largely replaced the fixed incremental pay systems introduced in the private sector during the 1970s'. Elected officials and public managers in many OECD countries support performance-related pay as an alternative to the traditional notion of seniority or job level to determine individual salaries. In the UK public sector, for example, PRP has been supported by successive governments as a mechanism to improve the efficiency of services – for example, within the civil service, and for school teachers. Evidence internationally is available to show that properly implemented schemes can contribute to improvements in public sector management. Nevertheless, there are problems with such schemes not least that there is a lack of rigorous evaluation which makes it difficult to determine the impact on efficiency (OECD, 1993).

How does it work?

Performance-related pay in practice can be seen as an extension of the performance and appraisal process. Where appraisal includes objective setting, then the determination of pay can follow from the setting of objectives. In other words, objectives are set for the individual member of staff and performance against them is linked to pay. How this operates is shown in Figure 14.1.

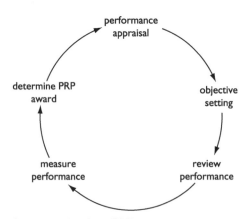

Figure 14.1 The performance-related pay (PRP) process

Once objectives have been set, the individual goes about meeting them. The supervisor monitors and helps the individual during the year, at the end of which there is a formal review of performance in the light of the objectives. The PRP award then reflects the extent to which objectives were met. This leads to setting fresh objectives for the next round, and the process begins again. For many employees, a system like that described has an intuitive appeal. They believe that it is unjust that two individuals should receive the same pay even though one is performing much better than the other, and they feel motivated by having clear objectives and standards against which they can measure their performance.

However, the experience with PRP is mixed and its transfer to the health sector has been associated with a range of problems. You will have learned in Chapters 12 and 13 that there is often a tension created in providing performance-related incentives to *individuals*, since this can preclude their ability to work towards wider organizational objectives. However, some argue that PRP, if applied to the right organization or system-wide needs, may enable individuals to work more for the benefit of the organization.

✎ Activity 14.1

1 Why are there problems in applying PRP to individual members of health care organizations?
2 What suggestions might you make as regards other options?

↻ Feedback

Some of the issues mentioned should be familiar to you from your reading of previous chapters in this book, others may not be. These are some of the points you may have identified:

- In health care, team contribution prevails over the contribution of individual members of staff.
- The power of professional organizations enables them to resist management initiatives.
- The agency relationship between health care professionals and patients can exclude and disadvantage employers.
- Employers try to retain insiders rather than recruit outsiders, even if they have to pay more. The authors suggest that in health services, doctors count as insiders and nurses as outsiders.

An alternative method of rewarding health care staff which avoids such problems might be to create compatible incentives and contracts at the level of health care teams (Bloor and Maynard, 1998). Thus, instead of giving individual doctors rewards for hitting service targets, the awards might be given to teams who are jointly rewarded. This has been partially applied in the new contract for general practitioners and other primary care professionals in England where, since April 2004, practice teams are rewarded based on the attainment of key quality and efficiency targets. Though this has yet to be evaluated, the team approach is designed to retain clinical freedom whilst curtailing inefficiency through internal monitoring by peers. The opportunity of bringing together staff with different skills (doctors, nurses, pharmacists and others) also moves in the direction of developing coherent service teams. As you saw in the last chapter, team-based working in health care is essential for managing quality across the supply chain.

Is there a theoretical justification for PRP in health services management?

The theoretical argument for PRP is often drawn from the concept of reward management that stems from classic neo-liberal economics. In other words, pay should be used rather than internal relativities to attract, motivate and reward key staff and that the focus should be more on the individual needs of managers to have flexibility to manage than to satisfy collective demands and requirements (Armstrong, 1993).

Expectancy theory would suggest that effort (input) is directly related to the achievement of performance and that such effort is only provided by individual reward (Vroom, 1964). In itself, expectancy theory says little about other motivations such as pay or job satisfaction, but assumes a link between pay and performance. However, it is clear from reviews of the subject that pay is but one factor influencing performance (Martin, 1994). Moreover, it is clear that organizations have faced a series of dilemmas in introducing PRP, the most important of which are that PRP tends not to reward team building and focuses too much on quantitative and measurable outputs ('bean-counting') rather than addressing the key issues of organizational performance.

Motivation and pay

The public sector literature shows that the greater reliance an organization places on financial incentives, the less doctors are willing to respond in the best interests of patients when not directly rewarded. In Le Grand's (2003) theory of public service motivation, for example, he postulates that the often 'knightly', or altruistic, nature of health service providers creates a highly complex relationship between pay and performance. Hence, for some, financial rewards may reinforce motivation towards the supply of care (what Le Grand terms *'crowding-in'*), but for others the pay incentive may actually erode motivations (*'crowding-out'*). The latter is particularly apt in health services since (as is often the case) such rewards have often been imposed in a system seeking to impose control over the traditional powers and freedoms of professionals. Since the motivations of those that deliver health services are complex and not purely motivated by 'knavish' self-interest or financial reward, the best management strategy is likely to be one that is more robust than a simple PRP mechanism.

It can be concluded from such evidence that, for PRP to work in health care, it has to be based on an objective rating scheme that deals with organizational outcomes (as well as activity), which appeals to both the 'knavish' and 'knightly' motivations of staff, and which provides the greatest opportunity for as many people in the organization to earn additional money.

Activity 14.2

The above debate has examined how performance-related pay may influence the motivation of staff. Thinking more broadly about the nursing profession in your own country:

1 What distinctive features of professions make performance measurements difficult?
2 Can PRP enable nursing to improve? If so, what do you think are the prerequisites needed to achieve this?
3 What do you think might be the key detrimental effects of PRP on motivation?

Feedback

1 Professions like nursing make performance measurements problematic since they are characterized by many features that are not directly measurable. As Martin (1994, p. 13) suggests, these might include:

- *Intangibility* – where the output of nurses cannot normally be seen, heard, tasted or felt before being consumed or purchased;
- *Inseparability* – where nurses and patients are inextricably interlinked;
- *Perishability* – where the service is consumed immediately and cannot be stored; and
- *Variability* – where the quality of the service depends on who is providing it and the quality of the interaction between producer and consumer.

2 It is sometimes argued that PRP can be effective if certain organizational character-istics are met. These include specific issues to do with the context in which services are provided, including:

- a supportive organizational culture in which the values of the organization and its staff are geared solely towards achieving performance;
- high trust relations, where employees and employers have the same objectives;
- a system with objective measurements and a willingness to accept performance ratings;
- staff that are competent in training and appraisal; and
- sufficient money available to provide the necessary financial incentives.

The nature of nursing does not lend itself well to PRP since the characteristics of the service are not so well defined and structured to meet these prerequisites.

3 There is some evidence that extrinsic rewards can erode the intrinsic motivation for the job. Simply getting people to chase money produces nothing except people chasing money. Moreover, whether change would really be engendered can be questioned since deep-seated nursing values might be less open to manipulation and change of their activities through managerially led PRP systems.

PRP and organizational performance

Performance measures that focus purely on efficiency may enable stability and procedural regularity but may be detrimental to quality, change and innovation. As you saw in the previous two chapters, in health services it is these latter activities that are arguably important measures of organizational performance. Health ser-vices managers, therefore, need to balance the attainment of efficiency goals with those aspects of quality which aim to meet the needs of patients.

In terms of PRP, and the use of financial incentives in general, it is clear that they need to be used in ways that impact on staff motivation without creating conflicts with other aims. For example, the use of end-of-year bonuses related to overall organizational performance might be argued to be a more socially coherent pay strategy than those based on individual activity.

When is PRP appropriate?

You may conclude from this chapter that *individualized* forms of PRP in health care have negative consequences in terms of the intrinsic motivations amongst staff, on teamworking and the size of the wage bill. You may also conclude that the appropriateness of PRP depends much on the organizational setting and the motivation of the post-holder.

It is important for you to consider the differences in motivation between professions that may apply when PRP is introduced. The following two quotations, the second from a well-known American songwriter, illustrate what has been called an *instrumental* work motivation.

I have no choice but to come to town because I need money. Why should a man undergo such hardship for any other reason? I must help my family. If that means working every day . . . I will do it. I cannot let my family suffer.

(Kenyan night-watchman, quoted in Blunt and Popoola, 1985)

Work five days a week, man, loading crates down on the dock,
I take my hard-earned money, and meet my girl down on the block.
Monday when the foreman blows time,
I already got Friday on my mind.

(Springsteen, 1980).

The research of Blunt and Popoola (1985) suggests that an instrumental motivation is found among low-status workers wherever jobs are scarce, whether in a low-income country or anywhere else. Workers value work principally for the material rewards it provides, which they can use to improve their lives outside work (like the docker in Springsteen's song). On the other hand, workers in high-status occupations, such as doctors and managers, are more likely to be *intrinsically* motivated; that is, they value work for itself rather than for the rewards that work offers, which they may take for granted when those rewards are sufficient.

Such differences between occupations need to be taken into account when designing pay systems, as do differences between organizations. The pay system that is appropriate for a small, growing private sector company will probably not suit a large, well-established organization in the public sector. However, you should be careful not to assume that a particular pay system is culturally appropriate simply because it is well established. Such a system is certainly *familiar*. It may or may not be *appropriate*. Moreover, you should be alert to the many other factors as well as pay which can affect staff motivation; for example, the extent to which staff are able to participate in decision-making and how much support they receive from their managers.

As Martin (1994) suggests, managers wishing to reward staff in health care organizations may be better advised to concentrate on refining locally relevant performance measures and consider group or organization-wide schemes over a prolonged period of time. Given the political and ideological support that PRP-based public sector reforms engenders in many countries as an approach to improving the technical efficiency of services, you may be faced with developing, managing and/or working within such systems in the future. You need to be aware of the potential problems and pitfalls to the approach.

Summary

You have seen that PRP is an alternative to fixed pay as it allows managers to align pay to performance and outcomes. The chapter has also discussed the problems of applying this concept to the health sector. Whether PRP is appropriate depends not only on the organizational setting but also on the work motivation, intrinsic or instrumental, that prevails among the professional groups. Reforming public-sector pay structures may be a little like redesigning the Pyramids, because pay structures, once established, are highly resistant to change.

References

Armstrong, M. (1993) *Managing Reward Systems*. Milton Keynes: Open University Press.
Armstrong, M. and Murlis, H. (1994) *Reward Management: A Handbook of Remuneration Strategy and Practice*. London: Kogan Page.
Bloor, K. and Maynard, A. (1998) Rewarding healthcare teams, *British Medical Journal*, 316: 369.
Blunt, P. and Popoola, O. (1985) *Personnel Management in Africa*. London: Longman.
Le Grand, J. (2003) *Motivation, Agency and Public Policy: Of Knights, Knaves, Queens and Pawns*. Oxford: Oxford University Press.
Martin, G. (1994) Performance-related pay in nursing: theory, practice and prospect, *Health Manpower Review*, 20(5): 10–17.
OECD (1993) *Private Pay for Public Work: Performance-Related Pay for Public Sector Managers*, Public Management Studies, OECD.
Vroom, V. (1964) *Work and Motivation*. New York: John Wiley.

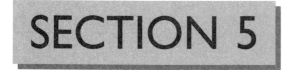

SECTION 5

Managing change

15 Determining strategic direction

Overview

In this and the next two chapters, you will learn about managing change. The best strategy for any organization depends on its mission, the resources and competencies it has at its disposal, and the environment in which it is operating. The strategic direction must be chosen by analysing these three elements and identifying what the organization must do to ensure 'strategic fit'. In this chapter, you will first consider the importance of creating a sense of organizational purpose in planning and achieving goals before assessing the role of strategic management and one common practical application – the SWOT analysis.

Learning objectives

After you have worked through this chapter you will be able to:

- **write a mission statement;**
- **describe the link between organizational mission and operational plans;**
- **define the terms 'strategic management', 'strategy' and 'strategic fit';**
- **describe a strategy analysis process.**

Key terms

Mission statement A statement expressing the purpose of an organization, department or individual. It should convey a clear sense of direction and form the basis for day-to-day decisions.

Strategic fit This occurs when the organization's goals (mission) are achievable given its resources and its environment.

Strategic management The process of analysis and decision-making that is concerned with ensuring strategic fit.

Superordinate goals The highest goals of an organization; fundamental desired outputs that enable managers to assess performance relative to its mission.

SWOT analysis The SWOT (strengths-weaknesses-opportunities-threats) analysis is a framework for analysing the fit between the mission, the resources and the environment. The purpose of a SWOT is to identify the critical issues an organization must address if it is to achieve its mission.

The need for a clear sense of purpose

All individuals need to reach agreement about what they are expected to achieve, and the same is true of an organization. Without that, organizations cannot ensure they have the skills and resources to achieve it, nor can they monitor their performance to assess how well they are doing. There are several key reasons for setting organizational goals, including:

- to promote legitimacy;
- to aid motivation amongst staff;
- to guide action;
- to provide a rationale for decision-making;
- to assess an organization's standard of performance.

Activity 15.1

From the list below, who do you think should be involved in defining your organization's mission. Put one tick for some involvement and two ticks for much involvement:

- the management board
- staff
- clients
- agencies which provide funds.

Feedback

Many researchers would suggest:

- the management board ✓✓
- staff ✓✓
- clients ✓
- agencies which provide funds.✓✓

Personal visions

The needs of patients, purchasers and funders must be taken into account when a health care provider draws up an organizational mission, but it is the personal visions of staff and leaders that are paramount. These personal visions of what can be achieved must be drawn together into a shared vision, which is then articulated as the organizational mission. The role of the person, or team, writing the mission is, therefore, to listen to the visions of others, to expose them to each other's visions and propose ideas which are as inclusive as possible.

This does not mean that missions have to be long and politically correct and state everyone's views. Some of the best are short and simple and would probably not have been phrased that way by most of the people consulted. However, they do recognize the sense and spirit of the statement.

Developing the mission statement

An organization's *mission* articulates its fundamental purpose in such a way that it both defines the business of the service or enterprise *and* articulates the values about the use of human, technical and financial resources. A well-framed *mission statement* provides a sense of purpose and establishes parameters that focus such efforts and resources. A good example from industry is as follows:

To passionately campaign for the protection of the environment, human and civil rights and against animal testing within the cosmetics and toiletries industry.

[The Body Shop]

Choosing a mission statement is not a one-time decision, since the purpose and needs of an organization will change over time. However, a key responsibility of senior managers is to articulate its fundamental values, goals and guiding concepts. Mission statements provide a sense of direction and are usually accompanied by a set of *superordinate goals* – the fundamental desired outputs stated in ways that enable managers to measure and assess specific performance targets.

Activity 15.2

Imagine you are the director of a publicly funded physiotherapy service. The key purpose of the service is to improve the mobility and independence of people in Old County. What do you think would be the key superordinate goals of the service?

Feedback

The following strategic goals might have been included on your list:

1 To offer advice on prevention, manipulation and exercise therapy to residents of Old County.

2 To convince potential patients and referrers (such as doctors) of the benefits of the services on offer.

3 To persuade funding agencies of the evidence of the efficiency of the services and of the mobility needs of Old County residents.

What makes a good mission statement?

Activity 15.3

Look at the following two mission statements. What do you think is right or wrong about each one?

1 A health clinic in a rural area

'We aim to provide services of the highest quality and to respect the choices and dignity of our clients. We recognize that our staff are our greatest asset.'

2   An audiology department in a hospital

'Our mission is to provide assessment and treatment services for patients with hearing problems.'

↻ Feedback

1 You may have said that you liked the sentiments of this statement – the concern for quality, respect for dignity and recognition of the importance of staff. However, the major problem with this statement is that it does not indicate the *purpose* of the services it provides. What is included is not made clear. Health services can have as their purpose the prevention and treatment of illness and/or they can be about the promotion of health. Health care organizations with these two different senses of purpose may behave quite differently so it is not enough to state the service you are offering; you must include the spirit or philosophy behind it. There are problems, too, in the use of phrases such as 'high quality' and 'respect for choices and dignity' in that they could mean different things to different people. They are woolly, not sufficiently clear.

2 You may have liked the brevity and clarity, and indeed this sentence should form part of the audiology department's mission statement. It does not, however, say *why* they are providing the assessment and treatment service. Is it so they can make money? Is it to maintain or increase the autonomy of people with hearing difficulties? The decisions taken within the service would be very different. Of course, it may be both, in which case both can be stated. It may also include the wishes of staff to pursue interesting and varied caseloads if that is important.

Translating goals into action

Goals are essential but they do not, of themselves, make things happen. They need to be translated into detailed plans. As Daft and Marcic (2000) suggest, there are five key characteristics of well-written goals:

1   specific and measurable
2   cover key result areas
3   challenging but realistic
4   defined time period
5   linked to rewards.

The fifth (linked to rewards) is much debated, particularly in the health sector. Indeed, many researchers have observed that rewards do not have to be linked directly to the goals, for reasons to do with the different motivational drivers which you learnt about in Chapter 14.

Strategic direction and management

There are three elements to take into account when identifying the most appropriate strategic direction for an organization:

1 the organization's mission (reviewed above);
2 the resources and competencies the organization has available;
3 the environment in which the organization is operating.

Thus, even organizations making the same products in the same industry (and therefore operating in the same environment and possibly having the same mission) will have different strategies because they will have different resources. Their staff will have different skills and enthusiasms; their production processes may be different; one may have a patent on a particular product or process; the other may have tied up all the supplies from a particular supplier.

Strategic management

Strategic management is the analysis and decision-making which is concerned with ensuring strategic fit. *Strategic fit* happens when the organization's goals (mission) are achievable given its resources and its environment. Strategic management can be divided into strategy formulation (deciding what the strategy should be) and strategy implementation (making it happen). In this chapter you are studying strategy formulation. Methods and techniques of implementation, in the context of change management, are examined in Chapters 16 and 17.

So, what is strategic management? You will find that in all textbooks on strategy there is constant reference to competitive advantage, or doing something better than other companies. For commercial companies, competitive advantage is important but it is not so important for publicly funded services. Making money is part of (only part of) the mission for commercial companies and so they must look for means of offering products which make money. This usually means doing something better than the competing companies. Health care organizations are rather different. Their aim is to meet the health care needs of clients. Some are commercial and for them competitive advantage is relevant. Some are not and yet strategic thinking is just as important for them as for the others. Their focus is not on competitive advantage but on maximizing the organization's ability to achieve its aims (mission).

Strategic analysis

The three elements of strategy are mission, resources and environment and managers are seeking to ensure that there is a good match between them (strategic fit). A strategic analysis must scrutinize all three elements and look at how they fit together. The framework most commonly used for this purpose is a SWOT analysis, so called because it is an acronym of its parts: Strengths, Weaknesses, Opportunities and Threats.

SWOT analyses

The SWOT analysis is about 40 years old and is used to identify priorities for action (Ansoff, 1965). A team or other sub-unit of an organization writes down its mission or purpose. Then, keeping this mission in mind, they then identify all their strengths and weaknesses and do the same for opportunities and threats. In some cases, they may be aided by a checklist of activities that need analysing (using a process such as PESTELI or the 7S model – techniques you will learn about in Chapter 17).

The main principle underlying SWOT is that internal and external factors must be considered simultaneously, when identifying aspects of an organization that need to be changed. Strengths and weaknesses are internal to the organization; opportunities and threats are external.

Activity 15.4

Imagine you are reviewing the strategic priorities for a local NGO whose mission is to provide accessible, affordable care to pregnant mothers and young children in a low-income country in order to reduce maternal mortality and improve the well-being of both mother and child. You have been approached by a medical officer who wishes the NGO to deliver this care on behalf of the government through a funded contract. What are the key questions in a SWOT analysis that the managers of the NGO should ask itself?

Feedback

For *strengths and weaknesses*, key generic questions might include:

1 What are the consequences of this offer? Will it help or hinder us in achieving our mission? If the factor does genuinely help the achievement of the mission (and only if the positive impact on the mission is convincing), then indeed it is a strength. Similarly if, but only if, it hinders achievement of the mission it is a weakness.

2 What are the causes of this strength (or weakness)?

For *opportunities and threats*, the questions would be slightly different:

1 What impact is this likely to have on us? Will it help or hinder us in achieving our mission? Again, only if the opportunity helps the team achieve the mission can it be considered such; even if it causes the world to be a nicer place but fails to support the team's ability to achieve its mission, it will not be an opportunity for these purposes.

2 What must we do to respond to this opportunity or threat? The analyst now reflects on the mission and all four components, paying particular attention to the causes of the strengths and weaknesses, and to the responses required to the opportunities and threats, and links together common threads into a set of priorities for the team to address.

The uses of SWOT

SWOT analysis is a ubiquitous feature of business strategy texts and courses. In a survey of 113 UK companies, Glaister and Falshaw (1999) found that SWOT was one of the most widely used strategic planning tools in current use across a range of sectors. In health services, SWOT has been used in a variety of settings, including: the voluntary community health movement in India (Sharma and Bhatia, 1996); sub-acute care services in the USA (Stahl, 1994); and public oral health services in Finland (Toivanen et al., 1999). These publications provide descriptions of how SWOT was used in particular settings and do not attempt to evaluate the relative value of the technique.

In a review of its use in 50 UK companies, Hill and Westbrook (1997) found that SWOT often resulted in over-long lists of factors, general and often meaningless descriptions, a failure to prioritize issues and no attempt to verify any conclusions. Further, they found that the outputs, once generated, were rarely used. However, such findings do not invalidate the use of SWOT. They do, however, reinforce the point that SWOT needs to be used carefully and with the end in mind rather than as a process in its own right.

Summary

You have seen how organizations and all the departments within them need a clear sense of purpose. Their mission should be a shared vision – a purpose which everyone in the organization can recognize and which allows them to contribute their own personal vision. The mission statement should include the purpose and the strategic goals. After strategic goals come tactical and operational goals. Strategic management can be divided into strategic formulation and strategic implementation. The SWOT analysis is a framework for analysing the fit between the mission, the resources and the environment. The purpose of a SWOT is to identify the critical issues an organization must address if it is to achieve its mission.

References

Ansoff, H. (1965) *Corporate Strategy: An Analytical Approach to Business Policy for Growth and Expansion*. New York: McGraw-Hill.

Daft, R. and Marcic, D. (2000) *Understanding Management*. London: Harcourt College. Publishers.

Glaister, K. and Falshaw, J. (1999) Strategic planning: still going strong? *Long Range Planning*, 32(1): 107–16.

Hill, T. and Westbrook, R. (1997) SWOT analysis: it's time for a product recall, *Long Range Planning*, 30(1): 46–52.

Sharma, M. and Bhatia, G. (1996) The voluntary community health movement in India: a strengths, weaknesses, opportunities and threats (SWOT) analysis, *Journal of Community Health*, 21(6): 453–64.

Snell, L. and Newble, D. (2000) Strategic planning in medical education: enhancing the learning environment for students in clinical settings, *Medical Education*, 34(10): 841–50.

Toivanen, T., Lahti, S. and Leino-Kilpi, H. (1999) Applicability of SWOT analysis for measuring quality of public oral health service as perceived by adult patients in Finland, *Community Dental Oral Epidemiology*, 27(5): 386–91.

16 | Change management

Overview

In this chapter you will learn about change management in health services including its key terms and concepts. Building on previous chapters, you will consider the role of HRM in offering an integrated approach to managing and developing people in the context of a changing public sector. An empirical model is developed that enables you to apply design criteria for using HRM in change management. In particular, you will focus on organizational culture and how this can be managed.

Learning objectives

By the end of this chapter you will be able to:

- **understand and describe what is meant by change management and its key concepts;**
- **demonstrate that an integrated HRM model can provide an empirical approach to change management;**
- **analyse possibilities for change management from the perspectives of organizational culture.**

Key terms

Continuous change Change that is ongoing, evolving and cumulative.

Developmental change Change that enhances or corrects existing aspects of an organization.

Emergent change Change that is apparently spontaneous and/or unplanned.

Episodic change Change that happens infrequently as an organization or system moves from one strategy to the next.

Person-oriented organizational culture A professional culture in which the organization has no intrinsic value beyond the growth, development and self-realization of its members.

Planned change Change that is a product of conscious reasoning and action.

Power-oriented organizational culture Attitudes tending towards aggression and exploitation within organizations that are autocratic and controlled from the top.

Role-oriented organizational culture A setting in which the correct response tends to be more highly valued than the effective one, within typically bureaucratic organizations that are slow to adapt to change.

Task-oriented organizational culture Achievement and effectiveness are valued above the demands of authority or procedure within organizations whose structure is adaptive to tasks or functions, and emphasis is placed on rapid and flexible response to change conditions.

Transformational change Change that is accepted by on organization as a norm so that a continuous improvement cycle of adaptation is developed.

Transitional change A purposeful strategy of change that is undertaken to achieve a desired state that is different from the current one.

Whole systems thinking An approach in which issues, forces and actions are not seen as isolated phenomena but part of a connected system of activity.

What is meant by change and change management?

The need for change, or reform, in the health services of any country is fundamental to the management process. Managers of services need to adapt processes in the face of many contextual changes such as the creation of new technologies, changing demographics and environmental pressures, rising demand and costs, and the imposition of different political ideologies in the way public services should be run. For health services to remain efficiently managed and to remain of appropriate quality and accessibility, the delivery of services must continually adapt to meet these changing contexts. So how does change occur?

Planned versus emergent change

Planned change is the result of a reasoned and deliberate set of actions by managers. However, change is often *emergent* – occurring naturally and in an unplanned fashion. Emergent change can happen when external factors (such as changes in the economy) or internal factors (such as the relative power of professional stakeholders) influence organizations in a way that is outside the control of the manager. Moreover, as Mintzberg (1989) argues, managers also make decisions on a daily basis and, whether planned or not, these can dictate the direction an organization takes.

Iles and Sutherland (2001) suggest that, this highlights two crucial elements in change management:

- the need to identify, explore and perhaps challenge the assumptions that underlie managerial decisions;
- an understanding that organizational change can be facilitated through planning but can never be fully isolated from the effects of serendipity and chance.

The central message in Iles and Sutherland's review of change management practices is that organizational change 'is not fixed or linear in nature but contains an important emergent element'.

Episodic versus continuous change

Another distinction to make about the nature of change is that it can be either *episodic* or *continuous*. Episodic change refers to intentional, planned and often radical change strategies. In contrast, continuous change is incremental and characterized by the natural adaptation of organizations over time in response to different stimuli. As a manager, the distinction is useful, since managers can capitalize on the natural change process by creating flexible systems with the ability to deal with everyday changes in organizational life – such as ambulances breaking down or the effects of a very cold winter on the health of the elderly.

Developmental, transitional and transformational change

Ackerman (1997) further distinguishes change by the extent of its scope. Hence, *developmental change* is incremental and enhances aspects of an organization – such as improving skills of staff through training and work experience. *Transitional change* is more episodic and managed, and has been subject to much examination. Lewin (1951) conceptualized a three-stage process involving:

- *unfreezing* the existing organizational equilibrium;
- *moving* to a new position;
- *refreezing* in a new equilibrium position.

Transformational change is the most radical in nature. The process involves a conscious effort to change the culture and assumptions of staff within organizations, often including major changes to structures and processes of management and delivery. These three perspectives on the nature of change are summarized in Figure 16.1.

Systems thinking and change

Have you ever heard of the phrase 'there is no such thing as a free lunch'? Or, 'every action has an opposite and equal reaction'? In both cases, the statements recognize that no action can happen in isolation and must have some form of knock-on effect elsewhere, and not necessarily in the intended direction.

Activity 16.1

Think about a major intervention that you, or your organization, has undertaken to bring about change to the way your organization functions.

1 To what extent did the intervention bring about the intended change?
2 Were there any unintended consequences of these actions, and were these positive or negative?
3 How might those designing the intervention be made more aware of its potential unintended consequences?

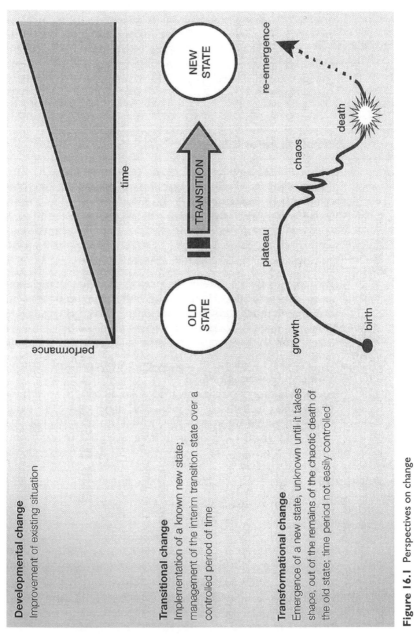

Developmental change
Improvement of existing situation

Transitional change
Implementation of a known new state; management of the interim transition state over a controlled period of time

Transformational change
Emergence of a new state, unknown until it takes shape, out of the remains of the chaotic death of the old state; time period not easily controlled

Figure 16.1 Perspectives on change

Source: Iles and Sutherland (2001), adapted from Ackerman (1997)

C **Feedback**

Whether or not the intervention you, or your organization, introduced was successful in bringing about intended changes, it is more than likely that a series of unintended side-effects were also produced. This is because the impact of change cannot usually be predicted in a linear fashion. Take the example of the deforestation of a tropical rainforest. The intended outcome may have been to develop a flourishing trade in lumber and hence economic growth. However, despite local environmental concerns, it was not recognized *at the outset* that such activity could lead to significant micro and macro climate changes.

Whole systems thinking

Whole systems thinking is now routinely used by managers and clinicians in many countries to reduce the potential of unintended adverse effects. The idea behind whole systems thinking in organizations originated from the 'ecological school' of engineering and manufacturing in the USA in the 1920s, a philosophy underpinned by adapting the laws of nature to a business environment. Hence, it was assumed that any activity within an ecosystem (organization) resulted in a range of influences and changes on other elements of the system.

The essence of *whole systems thinking* lies in seeing interrelationships rather than linear cause-and-effect chains. Thus, rather than breaking management practices and organizations into their component parts, systems thinking examines the properties that exist once the parts have been combined into a whole. Applied to change management, whole systems thinking highlights the following points:

* a system is made up of related and interdependent parts, so that any system must be viewed as a whole;
* a system cannot be considered in isolation from its environment;
* a system which is in equilibrium will change only if some energy is applied;
* players within the system have a view of that system's function and purpose, but these may be very different from each other (Iles and Sutherland, 2001).

✎ **Activity 16.2**

How relevant do you think whole systems thinking is to the management of health services? Think of some uses for the approach.

C **Feedback**

Within health services, whole systems thinking has widespread uses. For example, it might enable health and social care teams understand the need to work together to deliver seamless services to meet complex care needs; or it could be used to develop shared values and cultures within and between organizations to engender commitment and coherence.

The change management challenge

Undertaking change management to improve the delivery of health services faces a series of problems including changing environmental pressures; changing technologies; the complexity of organizational systems; the many competing views of stakeholders; and the potentially adverse impact of unforeseen or unintended consequences. As you will see in Chapter 17, no single change management strategy will fit all problems and all situations, but managers facing the challenge of managing change need to be adept at choosing the right tools for the circumstances they face.

The HRM model and change management

From previous chapters you have seen that the HRM model has been applied within organizations to cope with change and respond to demands in their external environments. However, it is also apparent that there is no single form of the HRM model, in terms of underlying values or criteria, for judging its effectiveness. In managing change you need to analyse your own organization's approach to HRM. This is to help you build any normative ideas of reform you may propose ('what ought to be') on an empirical picture of your organization ('what is').

Experience suggests that, in cases of successful organizational transformation, the *process* of working towards change is as important as the end results aimed for. In other words, an essential feature of organizational success in the face of environmental change is achieving new thresholds in how health care workers communicate, collaborate and learn together, and that these processes become explicitly valued in the organization's culture.

A systems model for organizational change

Table 16.1 provides a diagnostic framework which recognizes that the ability to achieve organizational change rests on actions within the political, cultural and learning systems of the organization as well as its technical systems. It adopts a systems approach for the diagnosis of change components based on Tichy (1985).

1 The *political system* concerns formal and informal configurations of power and influence, including access to and use of decision-making.
2 The *technical system* describes the arrangements combining human, technical and financial resources in production or service delivery.
3 The *cultural system* encompasses organizational values, including the differing beliefs, attitudes and behaviour of various subgroups, which are a critical component in designing change strategies.
4 The *learning system* (added to Tichy's original model) concerns how knowledge and skills are acquired and utilized at the individual, group and organizational levels. The overall model implies an open system in which internal systems are constantly attuned to external economic, political and cultural forces, and to each other.

Table 16.1 A systems basis for an empirical change model: key issues

	Overall strategy	Human resource strategy
Political system	Who determines mission and what should it be? How is coalitional behaviour around strategic decisions to be activated and judged?	How is succession in the organization to be handled? What rewards are appropriate to those exercising change responsibilities, and what sanctions for those not willing to cooperate with change leaders? What is the appropriate team-building activity? How can an appropriate empowerment of individuals/teams be undertaken?
Technical system	What is the current environment faced by the organization? What should constitute overall strategy and its fit with the resource base?- in terms of client satisfaction? How is performance to be improved?	What is the profile of the current workforce, its strengths and weaknesses? What are the competencies that need to be put in place to meet emergent demands? How are staff to be recruited and assigned roles? What performance appraisal system is appropriate? How are the required competencies to be developed?
Cultural system	What cultural values do the mission and strategy imply, and how different are these from those currently held by the workforce? Is it possible to make the necessary transformation given that cultural values are rooted in wider societal beliefs?	How is culture to be defined and measured in the organization? Can people be selected for jobs on the basis that they can build or reinforce the required culture? How can the appropriate culture be enhanced by training and development activities? Can people be rewarded for making the necessary transition to new values?
Learning system	How can learning be built into organizational activities to cope with the world of change? How can work systems be designed to give feedback to staff on their performance and on how they are learning to improve performance? What methods are available for individuals and teams to focus on their learning abilities? How can people become better learners?	What should constitute the primary means of individual and team competency building in the organization? How can managers foster a sense of the need for learning amongst employees? What learning resources should be available to further learning in the organization?

Source: Based on Tichy (1985).

Organizational culture

In any change management process it is essential that managers retain sensitivity to cultural issues in organizations. Schein's definition (1989) incorporates the process of cultural acquisition in organizations. He defines culture as:

a pattern of shared basic assumptions that the group learned as it solved its problems of external adaptation and internal integration, that has worked well enough to be considered valid and, therefore, to be taught to new members as the correct way to perceive, think, and feel in relation to those problems.

The common characteristics of culture in most definitions are:

*   its collective nature;
*   the sharing of norms, beliefs, values and assumptions;
*   their observable manifestations in behaviour.

In other words, culture represents the social reality of an organization; it can be considered the glue that binds members together. It contains various levels of learning and experience and is much more complex than its manifestations – observable in behaviour – would suggest.

Can culture be managed?

There are two opposing schools of thought on the role of organizational culture in change. On the one hand, culture is seen as a variable which can be created, amended or controlled by management. The management of culture becomes an explicit function through the communication of a mission, the presence of recognizable role models, and rewarded behaviour. The possibility also exists for more subliminal forms of control by the constant encoding of management style and other reinforcements of the required values. Influencing people's behaviour and beliefs in this way may imply manipulation or ideological control – potentially a more inclusive, pervasive and less identifiable form of control than traditional decision-making mechanisms, and one that raises critical questions.

On the other hand, culture can be regarded as something the organization *is* rather than something it *has* and that can be imported from outside the organization or created by management and passively accepted by staff. This perspective regards culture as the product of negotiated and shared symbols and meanings which emerge from social interaction over time. It cannot be created or manipulated by management but only described and interpreted. Schein (1989) refers to how basic assumptions, beliefs, values and meanings are shared unconsciously, in a taken-for-granted manner which makes them difficult to describe or grasp. Organizational culture is thus not amenable to management manipulation because it evolves through group learning. However, backing away from culture as a potential component in change, and seeing it as unmanageable, may lead to a lack of the introspection and self-analysis that successful organizations need, especially in a rapidly changing global environment.

Others argue that reality lies somewhere between these two propositions, particularly if it is accepted that culture operates at different levels in terms of its social and psychological effects. The possibility then arises of management influencing behaviour to meet organizational demands, whilst leaving deep-rooted values intact. Ogbonna (1992) suggests that this is how change management often works. Whilst managers promote values conducive to high performance, they do not necessarily wish to achieve this by covert manipulation, or they lack the ability to do so. Schein (1989) is more optimistic about changes in behaviour preceding and leading to changes in attitudes. He suggests that adopting and repeating new behaviours can lead to their becoming internalized as underlying values, but this inevitably takes time – and considerable time.

Schneider et al. (1990) support this in their distinction of organizational climate and organizational culture: *climate* consists of the current outlook of the workforce across diverse organizational activities, whilst *culture* represents beliefs and values at a deeper level of collective and individual psychology. They suggest that changing the climate through tangible policies, practices, procedures and routines will eventually impact on values and beliefs that guide employee behaviour. However, this type of change may affect only outward behaviour, with the risk that it may not go deep enough to create and sustain organizational transformation. Even when behavioural change is supported by the reinforcement of rewards or sanctions, the risk remains that such change will remain superficial – that it will not be sustained if these positive and negative incentives are removed. In addition, attempts to manage culture have to recognize that not all values may be shared by all members of the organization. There may be subcultures associated with different groups of staff, each of which has developed its own sense of what they are doing and why, and how people should relate to one another (Pettigrew, 1979).

Based on the above, you may ask yourself, to what extent do values, attitudes and beliefs play a role in your organization? Does management support the creation of a climate of positive attitudes towards work amongst staff? How concerned is management with issues of staff welfare and job satisfaction? Are HRM practices and procedures in place that enhance performance?

✏ Activity 16.3

Considering the recent history of your own organization:

1 Are employees' attitudes important in improving organizational performance? If so, what particular aspects of their attitudes?
2 Does the culture of your organization influence its performance?
3 Which are the most significant HRM practices for improving the performance of your organization?
4 How do managerial practices (other than the HRM ones you identified for the last question) impact on organizational performance? What are the most significant?

↻ Feedback

Four similar questions to the ones posed for your own organization were answered in a research project on 36 companies in the UK, with responses from 3500 staff (Patterson et al., 1997). The questions and some of the key findings are shown in Table 16.2.

Table 16.2 Organizational culture and performance

Question	Findings	Comment
1 Do employee attitudes predict company performance?	In relation to change in productivity, job satisfaction was identified as an important factor explaining 16 per cent of the variation between companies in their subsequent change in performance.	These results suggest that positive attitudes towards the work are an important predictor of performance. The more satisfied workers are with their jobs, the better the company's performance.
2 Does organizational culture significantly predict variation between companies in their performance and, if so, which aspects of culture appear most important?	Cultural factors accounted for some 10 per cent of the variation in profitability. In relation to change in productivity, the results were even more striking, explaining some 29 per cent of the variation between companies.	This is clear confirmation of the importance of organizational culture in relation to company performance. Concern for employee welfare was by far the most significant predictor.
3 Do human resource management practices explain variation between companies in profit and productivity?	The results reveal that (HRM) practices taken together explain 19 per cent of the variation between companies in change in profitability and 18 per cent in the variation of productivity. Job design and acquisition and development of skills (selection, induction, training and appraisal) explain a significant amount of the variation.	This is a most convincing demonstration of the link between people management and companies' performance.
4 Which managerial practices are most important in predicting company performance?	The authors assessed four areas, namely: •research and development •sophistication of technology •quality assurance •business strategy in their relation to performance.	Compared with these four domains, HRM practices were the most powerful predictors of change in company performance.

Source: Adapted from Patterson et al. (1997).

Note that these were private sector firms where performance was measured in terms of profitability and productivity.

Overall, these results clearly indicate the importance of people management practices in predicting company performance. This is ironic, given that the same research also demonstrated that emphasis on HRM is one of the most neglected areas of managerial practice within organizations. The implications are clear. But how can organizational culture be changed?

Culture in organizational change

The major issue at stake is not so much identifying the sorts of change required to improve organizational performance but how to achieve acceptance of change by those involved. This depends not just on a stated agreement with the new attitudes and behaviours but on internalizing them, which is more likely if the change process meets personal needs and enhances motivation and commitment to change.

Cultural engagement that employees experience can be characterized by two extremes:

negative reshaping <-> affinity with needs

An *affinity with needs* in cultural change increases the probability of acceptance of new organizational practices. To proceed without addressing the needs of stakeholders represents *negative reshaping* of culture with the risks of:

- unacceptably high levels of uncertainty and insecurity amongst staff;
- confusion amongst staff about the nature of proposed changes, leading to rumour and suspicion;
- uncompensated loss of informal status as change disrupts current status positions;
- incomplete preparation for new job roles as staff remain uneasy about having to learn new skills, take on different responsibilities, reach higher standards of performance or work with new colleagues in revised settings;
- staff feeling they are being hustled into change, because the transition period is too short or consultation has been inadequate, and hence resisting change.

Where previous experience of change has been negative because of inadequate consultation or serious disruption, the fear of new change is that much greater.

Harrison's model of organizational cultures

Harrison (1972) provides a useful model for investigating the disparity between the cultural orientation that employees are comfortable with and that imposed by the organization. He identifies four distinct organizational cultures.

1 *Power-oriented* organizations are autocratic and controlled from the top. There are few limits on the behaviour of the autocrat as long as he or she can maintain control of resources and can put down opposition. Relationships within the organization and with the environment tend to be aggressive and exploitative.
2 *Role-oriented* organizations are bureaucratic. Control is exercised and conflict minimized through systems of rules that assign rights and responsibilities. The correct response tends to be more highly valued than the effective one. Predictability of behaviour is high, and stability and respectability are often valued as much as or more than competence. Procedures for change tend to be cumbersome. The role-oriented organization is slow to adapt to change.
3 *Task-oriented* organizations weigh achievement and effectiveness above the demands of authority or procedure. Responsibility and authority are placed where the qualifications lie, and they may shift rapidly as the nature of the tasks of the organization change. Organizational structure is adaptive to tasks or

functions. Emphasis is placed on rapid and flexible organizational response to change conditions.

4 *Person-oriented* organizations exist to serve the needs of their members. The success of the organization is only a means to the growth, development and self-realization of the members. The organization has no intrinsic value beyond these goals, no super-ordinate goal, and it can be wound up when its usefulness to members ends. Responsibilities and tasks within the organization are assigned primarily according to members' own preferences and needs. Structure is loose and flexible, and management is through persuasion and mutual concern for the needs and values of other members.

Cultural difference manifests itself when two organizations or groups of people with different orientations come together in joint activities and projects. The greater the differences, the greater the potential for conflict, as representatives of two cultures find that their priorities, timescales and styles of working are different.

Summary

In this chapter you have learned about the nature of change and change management. Specifically, you have explored the application of the HRM model to the different stages of the life cycle of a health care organization. Emphasis was placed on organizational culture and its place in HRM-led change and you examined the Harrison model of organizational culture.

References

Ackerman, L. (1997) Development, transition or transformation: the question of change in organisations, in J. Hoy and D. Van Eynde (eds) *Organisation Development Classics*. San Francisco: Jossey Bass.

Harrison, R. (1972) Understanding your organization's characters, *Harvard Business Review*, 3, May–June: 119–28.

Iles, V. and Sutherland, K. (2001) *Managing Change in the NHS*, NCCSDO, London School of Hygiene and Tropical Medicine.

Lewin, K. (1951) *Field Theory in Social Science*. New York: Harper Row.

Mintzberg, H. (1989) *Mintzberg on Management: Inside our Strange World of Organizations*. Chicago: Free Press.

Ogbonna, E. (1992) Managing organizational culture: fantasy or reality, *Human Resource Management Journal*, 3(1): 42–54.

Patterson, M. O., West, M. A., Lawthorn, R. and Nickell, S. (1997) Impact of people management practices on business performance, *Issues in People Management*, 22, London: Institute of Personnel and Development.

Pettigrew, A. M. (1979) On studying organization culture, *Administrative Science Quarterly*, 24(2): 201–12.

Schein, E. H. (1989) *Organizational Culture and Leadership*. San Francisco: Jossey-Bass.

Schneider, B. (ed.) (1990) *Organizational Climate and Culture*. San Francisco: Jossey-Bass.

Tichy, N. (1985) Strategic approaches, in E. Huse and T. F. Cummings (eds) *Organization Development and Change*. St Paul: West Publishing.

17 Making change happen

Overview

In Chapter 15 you learned that a SWOT analysis allows you to identify the critical issues an organization must address if it is to identify strategic priorities. In Chapter 16, it was shown how planning and prioritizing change required an understanding of the nature of change itself and the predominant organizational culture. In this chapter, you will learn about some of the main tools and models that managers can use to make change happen.

Learning objectives

After you have worked through this chapter you will be better able to:

- **analyse your organization and its environment and identify the issues that must be addressed if it is to be successful in achieving its mission;**
- **understand underlying resistance to organizational change, the different models for achieving change and their relative effectiveness;**
- **understand frameworks for change and be able to design a change initiative to help deliver results.**

Key terms

7S model This model suggests that there are seven aspects of an organization that need to be in harmony with each other: strategy, structure, systems, staff, style, shared values and skills.

Business process re-engineering The fundamental rethinking and radical redesign of business processes to achieve dramatic improvements in performance such as cost, quality, service and speed.

Force field analysis Can be used to identify individual and environmental 'forces' that may help or hinder the successful implementation of change.

Organizational learning A transformational process that seeks to help organizations develop and use knowledge to change and improve themselves on an ongoing basis.

PESTELI A checklist for making sure all relevant aspects of the environment in which the organization is operating are considered.

Process modelling A way of understanding how a current situation works and providing a clear articulation of how a new one is to be different by visually capturing the dynamics of the situation so that they can be discussed with all those involved.

> **Soft systems methodology** Articulation of complex social processes in a participatory way, allowing people's viewpoints to be brought to light, challenged and tested.

How do managers understand and articulate strategic priorities?

You may have found yourself in a situation where you have tried to achieve change within a health care organization but come to the realization that the situation is so complex and dynamic that it is impossible to plan for every eventuality. This is not surprising since managers often have to address multiple priorities each of which compete for time and resources (for example, in achieving national targets versus addressing local or immediate needs). Living with such complexity is part of a manager's craft and many methodologies and tools have been created that allow managers to make better sense of their complex surroundings in order to develop a coherent strategic response.

Diagnostic tools: the 7S model

Many organizations in health services use diagnostic tools to assess where their organization sits in relation to what it is trying to achieve. They attempt to yield insights into the current strategic fit of an organization and are often used to justify change management programmes. A good example is the *7S model* (Figure 17.1), which suggests that there are seven criteria that need to harmonize with each other. As the name suggests, each criterion begins with the letter S as follows:

- *Strategy:* plan or course of action leading to the allocation of an organization's finite resources to reach identified goals;
- *Structure:* salient features of the organizational chart (for example, degree of hierarchy, presence of internal market, extent of centralization) and interconnections within the organization;
- *Systems:* procedures and routine processes, including how information moves around the organization;
- *Staff:* personnel categories within the organization such as nurses, doctors and technicians;
- *Style:* characterization of how managers behave in order to achieve the organization's goals;
- *Shared values:* the significant meanings or guiding concepts that an organization imbues in its members;
- *Skills:* distinctive capabilities of key personnel and the organization as a whole.

The 7S model can be used in two ways. First, strengths and weaknesses of an organization can be identified by considering the links between each of the criteria. Any criterion which harmonize with all the others can be thought of as a strength, any dissonances as a weakness. Second, the model highlights how a change made in any one of the criteria will have an impact on all of the others. Thus, if a planned change is to be effective, then changes in one criterion must be accompanied by complementary changes in the other. Note how this analysis reflects the philosophy of whole systems thinking examined in the previous chapter.

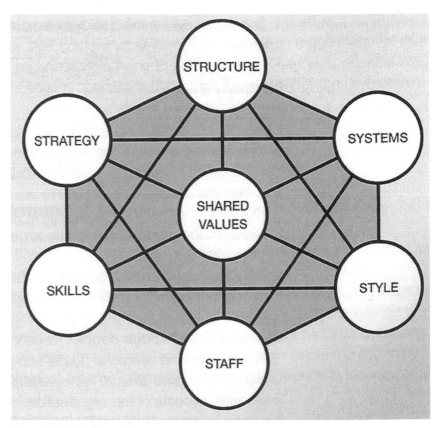

Figure 17.1 The 7S model
Source: Iles and Sutherland (2001), based on Peters and Waterman (1982)

✏️ Activity 17.1

Imagine two hospitals. One is a teaching hospital offering specialist care in complex cases to a population of 3 million people. The other is a general hospital offering good, reasonably priced care for routine cases to a local population of 200,000 people. Use the '7S' framework to describe some of the differences between them. As you do so, reflect on the need for the criteria to support each other.

↻ Feedback

Look at Table 17.1. This is not a definitive list but is intended to show linkages between the seven criteria. These are stereotypes of specialist and general hospitals and you will not find any hospital exactly like either of them. Can you see that the criteria link to each other in both cases? So, all are strengths even though they are very different from each other. If you switch any of the criteria so that, for example, the skills of the general hospital replaced the skills of the teaching hospital (or vice versa) then these skills stop being a strength and become a weakness. None of the criteria on their own is a strength or a weakness. It is the way each supports or impedes the other six that makes it an advantage (strength) or disadvantage (weakness).

Table 17.1 Understanding strategic linkages between two hospitals using the 7S framework

	Teaching hospital	General hospital
Aim	specialist care for complex cases	good, reasonably-priced care for routine cases
Strategy	high cost, differentiated by complexity of case	high throughput, low unit costs
Key systems	1 research, development and maintenance of leading-edge clinical skills 2 availability of specialist resources whenever needed 3 professionals encouraged to develop separate specialist skill bases	1 development of guidelines incorporating best practice (based on research at teaching hospital) 2 efficient scheduling of specialist resources, e.g. theatre time 3 good communication between professionals to speed throughput – some multi-tasking
Staff motivated by	1 development of knowledge and skills 2 intellectual challenges and complex clinical cases	1 care of patients (rather than clinical cases) 2 good relationships with other team members (good communication saves money)
Skills needed	1 research and development 2 specialist clinical skills	1 people skills 2 skills in utilizing resources effectively and efficiently 3 excellent skills in routine cases
Structure	functional structure	divisional structure
Style	deference to highly-skilled high-status individuals; more supportive than challenging: facilitation of challenge from other highly-skilled clinicians rather than from managers	participative and open but challenging as well as supportive
Culture	1 'We've got to be able to do it; there's no one else to refer to' 2 'We're pretty clever and important, especially me'	1 'We're all important here and views of other staff groups are essential' 2 'I'm OK, you're OK, we're all OK' 3 'Being challenged is fine, and I'm happy to challenge when I think it's necessary'

The 7S approach is attractive because of its dual emphasis on 'soft' (style, staff, skills and shared values) as well as the 'hard' organizational components (strategy, structure and systems). It can be criticized, however, as providing a one-sided perspective of organizational culture, focusing solely on the similarities that bind an organization and ignoring conflict and dissension.

PESTELI

PESTELI is a checklist for analysing the environment of an entire organization or part of one. The acronym stands for:

- *Political factors* – political forces and influences that may affect the performance of, or the options open to, the organization;
- *Economic influences* – the nature of the competition faced by the organization and the financial resources available within the economy;
- *Social trends* – demographic changes, trends in the way people live, work and think;
- *Technological innovations* – new approaches to tackling problems not necessarily confined to technical equipment – they can be novel ways of thinking or of organizing;
- *Ecological factors* – definition of the wider ecological system of which the organization is a part and consideration of how the organization interacts with it;
- *Legislative requirements* – which extend from employment law to environmental regulations;
- *Industry analysis* – a review of the attractiveness of the industry of which the organization forms a part.

Like the 7S model, this checklist can be used to analyse those factors in the environment helpful to the organization and those which may impede progress. PESTELI has too often been included as a stand-alone section in reports and not linked to any implications for organizational action (Iles and Sutherland, 2001). This can lead to considerable expenditure of time and energy for little benefit. There is, thus, a danger you need to be aware of that is common to all checklists – that of 'tick-boxing' without reference to the aims of the organization or to the change programme.

Soft systems methodology

Soft systems methodology (SSM) articulates complex social processes in a participatory way, allowing people's viewpoints to be brought to light, challenged and tested. SSM comprises the following stages (Figure 17.2):

1   Finding out about a problem and its causes from stakeholder, cultural and political perspectives, without attempting to impose a preconceived structure or to over-simplify the processes.
2   Articulating 'root definitions' of relevant systems – statements which encapsulate the main purpose, dynamics, inputs and outputs.
3   Debating the situation with those involved by depicting activities required to

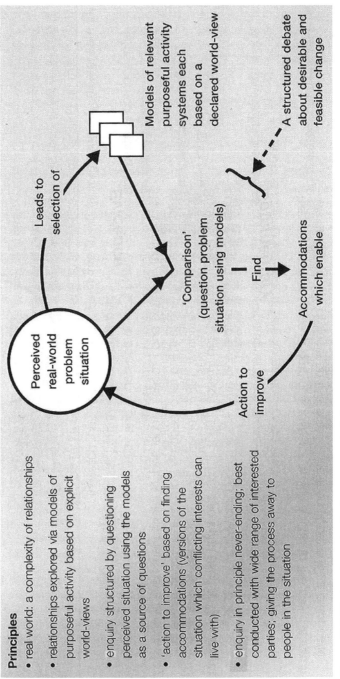

Principles

- real world: a complexity of relationships
- relationships explored via models of purposeful activity based on explicit world-views
- enquiry structured by questioning perceived situation using the models as a source of questions
- 'action to improve' based on finding accommodations (versions of the situation which conflicting interests can live with)
- enquiry in principle never-ending; best conducted with wide range of interested parties; giving the process away to people in the situation

Perceived real-world problem situation

Leads to selection of

Models of relevant purposeful activity systems each based on a declared world-view

A structured debate about desirable and feasible change

'Comparison' (question problem situation using models)

Find

Accommodations which enable

Action to improve

Figure 17.2 The learning cycle of soft systems methodology

Source: Iles and Sutherland (2001), based on Checkland and Scholes (1999)

achieve the root definitions, for example, through process flow charts or influence diagrams.

4 Comparing models with reality, by observation and discussion, and defining possible changes of structure, process and attitude.

5 Taking action to implement the changes.

In health care, SSM-based case studies have focused on a wide range of issues including simulations for resource allocation and planning, analysis of nurse management and activity, and the relocation of specialty services. However, there have been concerns raised about the time and cost implications of using SSM and whether organizational members can be motivated sufficiently to carry the process through to its conclusion (Iles and Sutherland, 2001).

Process modelling

One way of gaining clarification of different views and expectations of a process is to use process modelling. This is a way of increasing understanding of how the current situation works and provides a clear articulation of how the new one is to be different. It does this by capturing visually the dynamics of a situation so that they can be discussed with all those involved. Two examples of process modelling include *process flow* which represents diagrammatically all the stages involved in the completion of a particular process (see Figure 17.3 for an example) and the *theory of constraints*, which applies process modelling techniques to identify bottlenecks in organizational systems. In both cases, identifying the points at which systems 'fail' enable managers to identify key areas that need to change.

Understanding who and what can change

Understanding who and what to change requires a recognition that people – individuals and teams – are the key to lasting change in health service delivery. Early analysis of this issue can be found in Lewin's (1951) *force field* model. Force field analysis is based on the concept of forces, a term which refers to the perceptions of people in the organization about a particular factor and its influence. *Driving forces* are those forces which are attempting to push it in a particular direction. These forces tend to initiate change or keep it going. *Restraining forces* act to restrain or decrease the driving forces. A state of equilibrium is reached when the sum of the driving forces equals the sum of the restraining forces (Figure 17.4).

Lewin formulated three fundamental assertions about force fields and change:

1 Increasing the driving forces results in an increase in the resisting forces; the current equilibrium does not change but is maintained under increased tension.

2 Reducing resisting forces is preferable because it allows movement towards the desired state, without increasing tension.

3 Group norms are an important force in resisting and shaping organizational change.

A force field analysis can be used to identify actions that would enhance the successful implementation of change. Research supports Lewin's assertions that working to reduce the resisting forces is more effective than efforts to increase the driving ones.

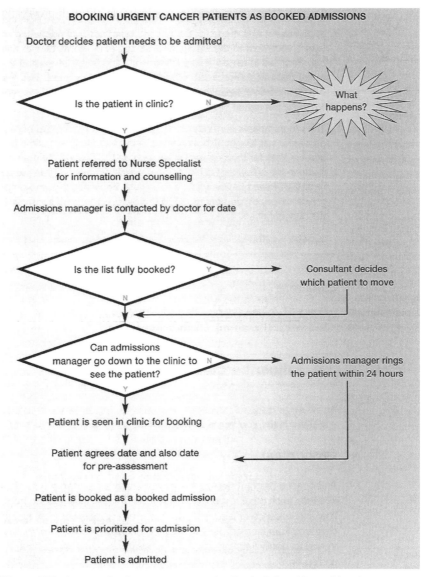

Figure 17.3 An example of a process map used at King's College Hospital, London

Source: Iles and Sutherland (2001)

The Wrecking Powers Game

The Wrecking Powers Game (adapted from Pedler et al., 1994) is a type of force field analysis which analyses the power of different stakeholders and their 'force' in the achievement or otherwise of organizational objectives.

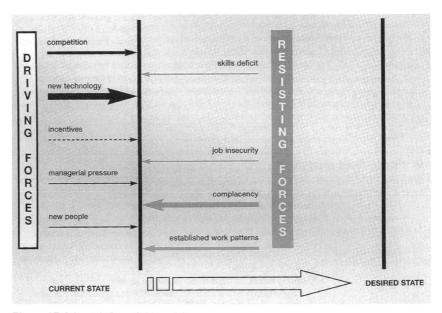

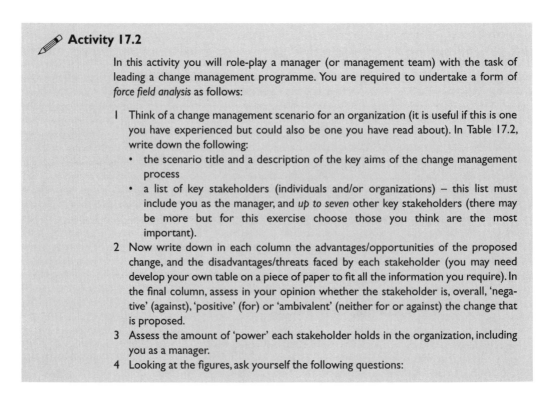

Figure 17.4 Lewin's force field model

Source: Iles and Sutherland (2001), based on Lewin (1951)

✏ Activity 17.2

In this activity you will role-play a manager (or management team) with the task of leading a change management programme. You are required to undertake a form of *force field analysis* as follows:

1 Think of a change management scenario for an organization (it is useful if this is one you have experienced but could also be one you have read about). In Table 17.2, write down the following:
   - the scenario title and a description of the key aims of the change management process
   - a list of key stakeholders (individuals and/or organizations) – this list must include you as the manager, and *up to seven* other key stakeholders (there may be more but for this exercise choose those you think are the most important).
2 Now write down in each column the advantages/opportunities of the proposed change, and the disadvantages/threats faced by each stakeholder (you may need develop your own table on a piece of paper to fit all the information you require). In the final column, assess in your opinion whether the stakeholder is, overall, 'negative' (against), 'positive' (for) or 'ambivalent' (neither for or against) the change that is proposed.
3 Assess the amount of 'power' each stakeholder holds in the organization, including you as a manager.
4 Looking at the figures, ask yourself the following questions:

- Is it obvious where the power lies?
- What *types* of power characterize those stakeholders you ranked highest?
- As a manager, what are the main strengths and weaknesses in terms of the power that you hold in the organization?

5 If there are stakeholders that you ranked as 'more powerful' than you as a manager, and who are resistant to change, mark these as 'key wrecking powers'. Develop a plan of action for dealing with these potential 'wrecking powers' in the organization.

Table 17.2 The Wrecking Power Game – a framework for analysing negative and positive stakeholders to the change process

Stakeholder	Key advantages and/ or opportunities of change to the stakeholder	Key disadvantages and/or threat of the change to the stakeholder	Attitude $(+, - \text{ or } =)$[1]	Power rating $(0 \text{ to } 5)$[2]	Wrecking power?
Manager of change			+		No

[1] + for positive, – for negative, = for ambivalent
[2] estimate level of power using the following power rating scale: 5 = very strong; 4 = strong; 3 = adequate; 2 = weak; 1 = very weak; 0 = desperate

Feedback

1 Lists of stakeholders will vary by scenario but your list might have included managers, professional groups, patients, funding agencies, local authorities, governments, NGOs, the voluntary sector and even the police or security forces.

2 Some stakeholders may have a lot to lose and others a lot to gain from the organizational change being considered. The analysis here enables the manager to map the *strength of opinions* amongst stakeholder groups both for and against the process. If you included patients in your analysis, you may have considered them to have weak levels of

influence – this is a common finding and reflects a malaise in health services generally at empowering and including patients in health services design.

3 Stakeholders marked as 'wrecking powers' are those the manager must address as a priority since their power reflects their importance to the functioning of the organization as a whole and without whose support the change is unlikely to succeed. Dominant 'wrecking powers' in health services are often those with entrenched professional or managerial interests. All other stakeholders marked as 'negative' or 'ambivalent' are still *potential* wrecking powers, since these stakeholders remain unconvinced, or unaware, of the mission and the consequences of the change being considered.

4 There are many key sources of power, such as:

- *Positional* – formal, hierarchical and status-related; when one person or group is 'higher' than another in the structure of an organization;
- *Resource* – mainly financial but also other valued resources such as access to key people and information; 'resource' power is often used to counter 'positional' power;
- *Knowledge and expertise* – possession of the technical ability or professional knowledge, such as by key clinicians, is power that is also often used to counter both 'positional' and 'resource' powers;
- *Personal influence* – is exerted in a wide variety of ways; medical leadership is often seen as more powerful to motivating change amongst health care staff than managerial leadership, but other factors include intellectual weight, trust and personal charm;
- *Networks* – useful to discover the 'insider information' of what is really happening in organizations below the surface;
- *Energy and stamina* – the power to survive and adapt through strength of persistence.

Managers in health services may or may not have resource powers and, more often than not, have to deal with many professional stakeholders with positional and expertise powers.

5 If you encountered few 'wrecking powers' then it may be that the change management process has a greater chance of success. Nonetheless, as you saw in Chapter 16, this does not mean that a manager can ignore those in an organization just because of their powerful position. If you encountered many 'wrecking powers' then making change happen becomes more problematic. Retain the list of steps you produced on how you would manage the change process for use later in Activity 17.4.

Organization-level change interventions

In Chapter 13, you learnt that total quality management (TQM) was a process directed at establishing an integrated organization to enable improvements in organizational performance and outputs. Evaluation of TQM suggests that the way it has been implemented has often been sub-optimal. Indeed, the evidence suggests that reluctance from staff, especially medical staff, has been a key reason for failure. As Berwick et al. (1992) observe:

. . . where TQM has been tried in hospitals so far doctors are often not effective on quality improvement teams. They arrive late or not at all to the meetings, they dominate when they are present; and they sometimes leap to solutions before the team has done its proper diagnostic work on the process.

Business process re-engineering (BPR) is a similar technique for corporate transformation that came to prominence in the early 1990s. BPR, a term coined by Hammer and Champy (1993), is defined as:

. . . the fundamental rethinking and radical redesign of business processes to achieve dramatic improvements in critical, contemporary measures of performance such as cost, quality, service and speed.

The steps involved in implementing BPR are as follows:

1 *Prepare the organization:* clarification and assessment of the organization's strategic context; specification of the organization's strategy and objectives; communication throughout the organization of reasons for and purpose of re-engineering.
2 *Fundamentally rethink the way that work gets done:* identify and analyse core business processes; define key performance objectives; design new processes. These tasks are the essence of re-engineering and are typically performed by a multi-professional team that is given considerable time and resources to accomplish them. New processes are designed according to the following guidelines (Hammer and Champy, 1993):

   • begin and end the process with the needs and wants of the customer
   • simplify the current process by combining or eliminating steps
   • attend to both technical and social aspects of the process
   • do not be constrained by past practice
   • identify the critical information required at each step
   • perform activities in their most natural order
   • assume the work gets done right the first time
   • listen to the people who do the work.

   An important activity in successful re-engineering efforts involves early wins to generate and sustain momentum.
3 *Restructure the organization* around the new business process.
4 *Implement new information and measurement systems* to reinforce change.

The essence of BPR is a process of *discontinuous thinking* encompassing a move away from linear, sequential thinking to a holistic perspective on change. This reflects the whole systems thinking philosophy outlined in the previous chapter. However, the evidence for the success of re-engineering processes in health services is mixed.

✎ Activity 17.3

What do you think are the key reasons why organization-level change management schemes often operate poorly in practice?

> ↻ **Feedback**
>
> Top-down and imposed processes of re-engineering often do not prove successful in professionally dominated health care organizations. For example, many studies suggest radical, revolutionary change is fundamentally incompatible with the traditions and cultures of those delivering health services. Given the complex factors that govern individual behaviours in health service organizations and systems, there are no easy ways to influence individual behaviour. However, it is true that applying redesign techniques needs both bottom-up and top-down commitment if it is to succeed.

Making change happen

Successful change hardly ever follows a simple pattern of thinking followed by doing. Instead, thinking informs doing and doing informs thinking throughout the process in an *iterative* way. The most influential organizational development models in health services use this system of continuous learning to aid the transformation process.

Organizational learning

Organizational learning is a transformational process which seeks to help organizations develop and use knowledge to change and improve themselves on an ongoing basis. Argyris and Schön (1978) describe three levels of learning that may occur in organizations:

1 *Single-loop learning:* adaptive learning, which focuses on how to improve the status quo. Involving incremental change, it narrows the gaps between desired and actual conditions. Single-loop learning is the most prevalent form of learning in organizations.
2 *Double-loop learning:* generative learning, aimed at changing the status quo; members learn how to change the existing assumptions and conditions within which single-loop learning operates. This learning can lead to transformational change.
3 *Deutero-learning:* learning how to learn. Learning is directed at the learning process itself and seeks to improve both single- and double-loop learning.

Argyris and Schön suggest that most individuals appear to operate within their organizational context according to the following rules:

- Strive to be in unilateral control.
- Minimize losing and maximize winning.
- Minimize the expression of negative feelings.
- Be rational.

They observed that these rules often govern behaviour and are enforced through a set of behavioural strategies such as:

- advocating your own views without encouraging enquiry – hence, remaining in unilateral control and hopefully winning; and

- unilaterally saving face – your own and other people's – hence, minimizing upsetting others or making them defensive.

These rules and strategies underpin what is known as *model I theory*. Conforming to model I often leads to defensiveness and 'learning disabilities' such as withholding information and feelings, competition and rivalry and little public testing of assumptions about organizational processes and performance. A more effective approach, called model II, is based on values promoting valid information, free and informed choice, internal commitment to the choice and continuous assessment of its implementation. This results in minimal defensiveness with greater openness to information and feedback.

Organizational learning interventions are aimed at helping secure a change from model I to model II thinking in organizational members. A *learning organization* is thus characterized by continuous emergent change driven by single-loop, double-loop and deutero-learning processes. In order to achieve a continuous cycle of learning and change, Senge (1990) suggests that a learning organization is founded upon five disciplines:

1 *Personal mastery:* the discipline of continually clarifying and deepening personal vision, of focusing energies, of developing patience and of seeing reality objectively.
2 *Mental models:* the discipline of working with mental models allows individuals to unearth the assumptions and generalizations that influence their understanding of the world and shape how action is taken.
3 *Building shared vision:* involves unearthing 'shared pictures of the future' that foster genuine commitment and enrolment rather than compliance, encouraging people to excel and learn.
4 *Team learning:* builds the capacity of team members to suspend assumptions and enter into genuine thinking together. It also involves learning how to recognize patterns of interaction in teams, such as defensiveness, that undermine learning.
5 *Systems thinking:* the 'fifth discipline' integrates the other four, fusing them into a coherent body of theory and practice.

The concept of the learning organization is increasingly popular as organizations, subjected to exhortations to become more adaptable and responsive to change, attempt to develop structures and systems that nurture innovation (Peters and Waterman, 1982; Senge, 1990). However, there is little hard evidence of the effect of the theory of organizational learning in practice.

Why organizations resist change

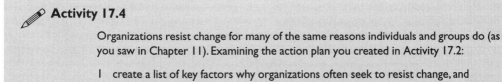

✎ Activity 17.4

Organizations resist change for many of the same reasons individuals and groups do (as you saw in Chapter 11). Examining the action plan you created in Activity 17.2:

1 create a list of key factors why organizations often seek to resist change, and
2 describe the methods by which you might seek to deal with resistance to change.

↻ **Feedback**

1 There are many forces inside an organization that create resistance to change. Bloisi et al. (2003) identify these factors (but your list may legitimately have many others):

- *Power maintenance* – changes in direction often shift authority and control and change the balance of power. Thus, professionals may seek to limit the imposition of new governance procedures; managers may seek to limit the creation of self-managed teams.
- *Structural stability* – organizations often condition the way individuals perform by, for example, creating jobs with specific roles and predictable tasks. As you saw in Chapter 16, a change in any one part of a system will have effects on others that may be regarded as both uncomfortable and acceptable.
- *Organizational culture* – you also saw in Chapter 16 discussed how organizational culture establishes values and expectations. When established assumptions are challenged, members may resist change.
- *Group norms* – groups within organizations can develop their own norms to promote desirable behaviour. Such groups, if highly cohesive, may resist change even if the change is seemingly beneficial.
- *Functional suboptimization* – functional units (such as clinical specialties and departments within a large general hospital) often work like independent fiefdoms and tend to think of themselves first before the organization as a whole. They may support changes that enhance their own welfare but will resist ones that reduce it.

2 Potential strategies to enable change include:

- *education and communication* to help people learn the reasons for change, and hence minimize resistance;
- *participation and involvement* to encourage people to help design and implement the change, thus reducing uncertainty and promoting ownership;
- *facilitation and support* to help people adapt to a new environment, such as through training, counselling and written guidance;
- *negotiation and agreement* through offering incentives for acceptance of the change such as job retention, pay awards, or opportunities for self-improvement;
- *coercion* – using authority and threat of negative incentives for non-compliance (such as reduced salaries, fewer benefits or even dismissal).

Evaluating and learning the lessons of change

One of the most important components in any change management programme is often neglected – *evaluating* the change. Without evaluation, learning can be lost to both organizations and to the individuals within them. The following review and learning questions should be part of the change management design (Iles, 1997):

1 Reviewing the change:

- Did the change achieve its objectives?
- How closely did it mirror the plan, and how did it differ?
- Why?

- How did the different stakeholders feel about the change?
- Is there anything more you can do to facilitate change of stakeholder views?

2 Learning for next time:

- What would you do differently another time?
- Why?
- How?

Finally, it is useful to remember that there is no right or wrong answer in managing change. Whether your organization or team responds to change depends on your ability to analyse the situation; to define (organizational) goals; to identify obstacles and facilitating factors in achieving the goals; and to deploy your resources tactically as a result. To manage change effectively, developing some of the managerial skills highlighted in the last three chapters and heeding the lessons they provide should be important to you as a manager of health services.

Summary

In this chapter you have learned how to understand the strategic priorities for an organization, including the potential need for change, through a range of diagnostic models. You also saw who and what to change through the adoption of force field analyses including an assessment of process re-engineering models, the need for the development of a learning organization and the potential resistance to change that is likely to be encountered. Finally, you learnt that evaluation of the change management process is essential in managing change.

References

Argyris, C. and Schön, D. (1978) *Organisational Learning: A Theory of Action Perspective*. Reading, Mass: Addison-Wesley.

Berwick, D., Enthoven, A. and Bunker, J. P. (1992) Quality management in the NHS: the doctor's role, *British Medical Journal*, 304: 235–9 and 304–8.

Bloisi, W., Cook, C. and Hunsaker, P. (2003) *Management and Organisational Behaviour*. London: McGraw-Hill.

Checkland, P. and Scholes, J. (1999) *Soft Systems Methodology in Action*. Chichester: Wiley.

Hammer, M. and Champy, J. (1993) *Reengineering the Corporation: A Manifesto for Business Revolution*. London: Nicholas Brealey.

Iles, V. (1997) *Really Managing Health Care*. Buckingham: Open University Press.

Iles, V. and Sutherland, K. (2001) *Managing Change in the NHS*, NCCSDO, London School of Hygiene and Tropical Medicine.

Lewin, K. (1951) *Field Theory in Social Science*. New York: Harper Row.

Pedler, M., Burgoyne, J. and Boydell, T. (1994) *A Manager's Guide to Self Development*. McGraw Hill.

Peters, T. and Waterman, R. (1982) *In Search of Excellence*. New York: Harper and Row.

Senge, P. (1990) *The Fifth Discipline: The Art and Practice of the Learning Organisation*. London: Doubleday/Century Business.

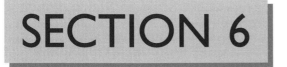

SECTION 6

The leadership role of managers

18 Management and leadership

Overview

It has become common in the management literature since the 1990s to draw a distinction between managers and leaders. However, leadership is an important managerial quality and you will have encountered elements of effective leadership in previous chapters on managing people and managing change. In this chapter you will learn more about the nature of leadership and the approaches to leadership you may wish to adopt.

Learning objectives

After working through this chapter you will be able to:

- understand the nature of leadership;
- describe the types of power available to a manager in health care;
- discuss a number of theories about the nature of leadership;
- devise a list of the qualities you believe an effective leader should possess.

Key terms

Coercive power Power to punish or to withhold rewards.

Empowerment The development of decision-making abilities amongst people at all levels in the organization.

Expert power Power resulting from specialist skills or knowledge.

Leadership A relationship through which one person influences the behaviour and actions of other people.

Legitimate power Power given by an organization, or by a statutory framework, to tell subordinates what to do. Subordinates accept this as legitimate.

Personal power Power arising from personality and behaviour. This includes expert and referent power.

Position power Power people have because of the position they hold in an organization. It includes legitimate, reward and coercive power.

Referent power Power that comes from personality characteristics that command identification, respect or admiration.

Reward power Power resulting from the ability to give rewards.

The nature of leadership

Activity 18.1

Leaders have a range of personal qualities that can make them more (or less) effective. Write down the names of two or three leaders you consider to be particularly effective (not necessarily in the health field) and set out the qualities that you think make them effective leaders. Compile a similar list for the names and qualities of two or three leaders that you think are ineffective. Is there one style of effective leadership that emerges?

Feedback

There are many ways to interpret what is and what is not effective leadership. In your lists, you may have written words such as authority, trust, charisma, wisdom, power, empathy and many others. This is because leadership is an abstract concept with different types of leaders appealing to different people. As Handy (1993, p. 14) reflects, 'finding a definitive solution to the leadership problem has proved to be another endless quest for the Holy Grail in organizational theory'.

Leadership and management

Good leadership is important since it helps to develop teamwork and the integration of individual and group goals. Whilst the role of managers is concerned primarily with the coordination of people working within organizations, leadership has a broader context and relates more to the quality of a person within a job, rather than the job itself.

Activity 18.2

1 What do you think are the key differences between leaders and managers?
2 How might you define managerial leadership?

C Feedback

1 Leadership is more about providing inspiration, whilst management is more about coordinating activities and making decisions. Compare your thoughts with those of Zaleznik (1977):

- managers tend to adopt impersonal attitudes towards goals whilst leaders adopt a more personal and active attitude;
- in order to get people to accept solutions, managers must coordinate and balance conflicting stakeholder views (see Chapter 11) – leaders create an overall environment or context that enthuses people to work collectively;
- in health care especially, good leaders tend to provide empathy towards people whereas managers are less emotionally involved;
- managers tend to regulate existing activity, leaders seek opportunities for change.

2 Despite these differences, you probably will have felt that leadership and management roles in health care organizations overlap. A common view is that for managers to do a job effectively they require significant leadership capabilities.

Leadership and power

Within an organization, leadership influence will be dependent on the type of power you can exercise over others. Mullins (1999) identifies three main sources of positional power related to leadership:

1 *Reward power* based on the perception that a leader can directly reward those who comply with directives (such as pay, promotion or praise).
2 *Legitimate power* based on the perception that a leader has the right to wield power which is based on authority and hierarchical position.
3 *Coercive power* based on fear and the perception that a leader can punish or bring about undesirable outcomes for those who do not comply with directives (such as withholding pay, withdrawing support or even dismissal).

✎ Activity 18.3

1 Think of your own organization and the managers within it. Do you agree that a manager's position gives him or her the power to reward or punish subordinates in order to influence their behaviour?
2 Write in Table 18.1 the forms of positional power you or your manager has in your own organization.

Table 18.1 Examples of positional power in your organization

Forms of positional power	Examples of my use of this form of power within my organization	Who in my organization exerts this kind of power?
Legitimate power		
Reward power		
Coercive power		

↻ Feedback

Many of the powers available to managers in other industries are not available to managers in health care. There are many reasons for this, including the status accorded to many health care professionals (especially doctors), the complexity of the technology, and the privacy of the relationship between professional and patient. You may well have found that although you have some legitimate power, there are important areas of work where you have little. You do not have the power to tell one of your staff exactly what to say to a patient, and would have only indirect ways of knowing if they had. In large bureaucracies, which health care organizations often are, reward systems are centralized, often negotiated for entire professions, and the individual manager has little input. Similarly the opportunity for use of coercive power is limited.

Personal power

Effective leadership in health care organizations is often based more on *personal power* than on positional power, since the former is often more effective in engendering belief and commitment. Mullins (1999) identifies two distinct forms of personal power:

1 *Referent power* based on the degree of *identification* with a leader due to their personal charm or charisma. Charismatic leadership, based on esteem and respect, is often found amongst networks of health care professionals where no single managerial authority exists.
2 *Expert power* based on the perception that the leader is the expert in his or her field and provides credibility and knowledge. Expert power is often limited to well-defined medical specialisms, or to expert managerial tasks (such as personnel management or systems analysis).

Building and using managerial power

There are no set rules for how managers should exert power and leadership over others. Indeed, the five sources of leadership power described above are inter-related and the use of one (such as coercive) may significantly impact on your ability as a manager to wield another (such as referent).

✐ Activity 18.4

Examine each of the five sources of leadership power. In Table 18.2, write down for each source of power at least three strategies you might use to increase and maintain that form of power and think of at least three ways in which that power might be employed most effectively.

Table 18.2 Strategies to increase and employ different types of power

Give three ways in which you could increase and maintain this form of power.	Give examples of how you would use this power effectively.
Reward power	
1.	1.
2.	2.
3.	3.
Legitimate power	
1.	1.
2.	2.
3.	3.
Coercive power	
1.	1.
2.	2.
3.	3.
Referent power	
1.	1.
2.	2.
3.	3.
Expert power	
1.	1.
2.	2.
3.	3.

↺ **Feedback**

Yukl (1989) examined the question of developing a set of guidelines on how to build and maintain power, and how to use it effectively to influence others. Compare your answer with that of Yukl reproduced in Table 18.3.

Table 18.3 Yukl's guidelines on how to build and maintain power in organizations

How to increase and maintain power	How to use power effectively
Reward power	
• discover what people need and want	• offer desirable rewards
• gain more control over rewards	• offer fair and ethical rewards
• ensure people know you control rewards	• explain criteria for getting rewards
• don't promise more than you can deliver	• provide rewards when promised
• don't use rewards in a manipulative way	• use rewards symbolically to reinforce
• avoid complex, mechanical incentives	desirable behaviour
• don't use rewards for personal benefit	
Legitimate power	
• gain more formal authority	• make polite, clear requests
• use symbols of authority	• explain the reasons for the request
• get people to acknowledge authority	• don't exceed your authority

Table 18.3 *contd*

How to increase and maintain power	How to use power effectively
• exercise authority regularly • give orders via proper channels • back up authority with coercive powers	• verify authority if necessary • be sensitive to concerns • follow up to verify compliance and insist on compliance if appropriate
Coercive power • identify credible penalties to deter unacceptable behaviour • gain authority to use punishments • don't make rash threats • don't use coercion in a manipulative way • use only legitimate punishments • punishments to fit the infraction • don't use coercion for personal gain	• inform target of rules and penalties • give ample prior warning • understand situation before punishing • remain helpful, not hostile • encourage improvement, not punishment • ask target for ways to improve • administer discipline in private
Referent power • show acceptance of positive regard • act supportive and helpful • keep promises • don't manipulate • make self-sacrifices to show concern • use sincere forms of ingratiation	• use personal appeals when necessary • indicate that a request is important to you • don't ask for a personal favour that is excessive or taking advantage • be a role model
Expert power • gain more relative knowledge • keep informed of technical matters • develop exclusive sources of information • use symbols to verify expertise • demonstrate competency • don't make rash judgements • don't lie or misrepresent facts	• explain the reasons for a request or proposal • explain why it is important • provide evidence that a proposal will be successful • listen to concerns • show respect (don't be arrogant) • act confidently and decisively

Source: Adapted from Yukl (1989)

Empowerment

For the reasons mentioned above, the amount of positional power available to health care managers is limited. Empowerment is therefore very important. It is almost the only way in which health care will be managed. It must not be seen, however, as a means for senior managers to opt out of unpleasant decisions, whilst retaining the pleasant ones.

Activity 18.5

How could the senior managers in your organization not simply wield power but also give it away to people who can get jobs done? Give three suggestions.

C **Feedback**

Suggestions you may have made include:

- devolving budgets to the lowest possible level;
- letting decisions be made by the people most closely involved;
- consulting people throughout the organization about any major changes, before they are made.

Personal qualities required in managers

The profile of personal qualities required varies with the positions a manager occupies in the health system. It makes a difference whether you work at chief executive officer level of a non-governmental organization, a multilateral agency, a health insurance company, a ministry of health, or a health care provider. The following activity enables you to compare the profile of a health care manager with your own qualities.

✎ **Activity 18.5**

1   Which of the qualities listed in Table 18.4 do you think a health care manager should have? Put a tick against them in column 2. In columns 3, 4 and 5 reflect on the

Table 18.4 Profile of personal qualities

Qualities	A health care manager should possess this quality	This quality is required for my role	I already possess this quality	I need to develop this quality
visionary				
rational				
passionate				
consulting				
creative				
persistent				
flexible				
problem-solving				
inspiring				
tough-minded				
innovative				
analytical				
courageous				
structured				
imaginative				
deliberate				
experimental				
authoritative				
initiates change				
stabilizing				
personal power				
position power				

qualities required for your own role in the health system. Depending on your position these may be different from or similar to those you have assigned to an ideal health care manager.

2 Place a tick in column 3 alongside those qualities that are necessary in your position.

3 Now, focusing on those qualities you have identified as necessary, to help you decide which of these qualities you need to develop, place a tick in column 4 against those qualities you believe you already possess. (You may like to discuss this with a friend.) Finally place ticks in column 5 to indicate those qualities you need to develop. This column can now form the basis for some personal development goals.

Feedback

Most health care services require people who combine many of these qualities. Some of the most important qualities:

- passionate (about quality of care);
- creative, flexible and innovative (about means of providing it);
- courageous (in maintaining integrity with staff and clients);
- imaginative and experimental (in the sense of being creative and rather than in the taking of large risks);
- rational, tough-minded, structured, problem-solving and analytical (in other words, able to think clearly and analyse carefully and objectively);
- consulting, persistent and stabilizing (important in the achievement of empowerment).

The following are less important but may be relevant in other settings of the health system:

- visionary
- inspiring
- deliberate
- authoritative.

Perhaps the most important quality of all has been omitted from both of these lists: that of *empathy*.

Summary

You have seen that the distinction between managers and leaders is less relevant in health care than in other industries. This is because the forms of power available to senior staff in health care are different from those in other industries. In particular, there is less legitimate power, reward power and coercive power. If a health care organization is to meet the needs of its patients then its senior staff must have some of the qualities of good managers and some of good leaders. They must also empower staff at all levels in the organization to take responsibility for an appropriate level of decision-making.

References

Handy, C. (1993) *Understanding Organizations*. London: Penguin, 4th edn.

Mullins, L.J. (1999) *Management and Organizational Behaviour*. London: Financial Times Pitman Publishing, 5th edn.

Yukl, G. (1989) *Leadership in Organizations*. London: Prentice-Hall International, 3rd edn.

Zaleznik, A. (1977) 'Managers and leaders: are they different?' *Havard Business Review*, May-June: 67–78.

19 Approaches to successful leadership

Overview

As you have seen in the previous chapter, health care managers are also leaders. In this chapter, you will learn about the different schools of thought about what it is that makes a leader successful. It shows how the different styles of leadership you adopt can have a significant impact on the motivation of staff in meeting organizational goals.

Learning objectives

After working through this chapter you will be able to:

- discuss different theories of leadership;
- analyse organizational settings and suggest an appropriate leadership style;
- consider the organizational setting in which your own leadership style is likely to be successful;
- understand how and why adapting your leadership style is essential in dealing with different stakeholders and situations that arise when managing health services.

Key terms

Autocratic leadership Leaders make decisions on behalf of their staff.

Behavioural approaches Theories that suggest that it is not personality but particular behaviours which determine whether or not a leader is successful.

Democratic (participative) leadership Leaders involve their staff in making decisions.

Trait theories Theories that suggest that leaders with certain personality traits will be more successful than others.

Theories of leadership

Leadership traits

Leadership traits are those distinguishing personal characteristics that make a leader successful. *Trait theories* assume that leaders are born and not made, and much research has been devoted to identifying the personality traits common to successful leaders. Hellriegel and colleagues (1998) identified four traits common to most (if not all) successful leaders:

- *intelligence* – a leader being in some way superior to followers;
- *maturity* – including a breadth of wisdom and interests;
- *motivational* – a high degree of inner drive for achievement;
- *people-centred* – the ability to respect and work well with others.

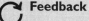 **Activity 19.1**

From your understanding of leadership and management gained in Chapter 18, what do you think are the key limitations to trait theories of leadership?

Feedback

The approach is limited because it is characterized by subjective judgements of what is a good leader and because the list of traits can be very long. It also does not help inform the development of future leaders, or the application of leadership skills. The traits approach has largely been discarded in the study of leadership.

Leadership behavioural theory

Leadership behavioural theories differ from trait theories since they suggest that it is not personality but particular behaviours that determine whether or not a leader is successful. One of the best-known works in this field is the Ohio State Leadership Study that examined the nature of different leadership styles on group perform-ance (Fleishman, 1974). Questionnaires were used across a range of different organizations and in a variety of situations, in which a list of descriptions relating to leadership behaviour were used. Results indicated two major dimensions of leadership behaviour:

1 *Consideration*, in which the leader establishes trust and respect through close empathetic communication with individuals and teams; and
2 *Structure*, reflecting the way a leader defines how the groups should organize themselves to achieve goals.

A key issue here is the extent to which these two behavioural types are combined. As Mullins (1999) suggests, *employee-centred* approaches (based on consideration) might be more effective in leadership than *production-centred* ones (based on structure).

Leadership styles

Leadership style is the way in which the functions of leadership are carried out. In other words, the way in which you as a leader in a health care organization behave towards different staff members. There are many dimensions to describing such behaviour – such as facilitative, dictatorial, unitary, bureaucratic, charismatic, consultative and participative – though Mullins suggests a broad classification based on three styles:

1 *Autocratic*, where power lies with the manager and the manager alone makes decisions, determines policy and controls rewards and punishments;
2 *Democratic*, where the focus of power lies in the group as a whole, so leaders must function in a consultative or participative manner;
3 *Laissez-faire*, where a leader observes that an individual or group works well on their own. In this style, a conscious decision is made to free members from managerial interference but, in the same vein, managers must be careful not to *abdicate* from their responsibilities.

The Blake and Mouton leadership grid

Blake and Mouton (1985) developed a leadership grid based on a combination of concern for production and a concern for people (Figure 19.1). The scale for each component moves from one (low) to nine (high). Five leadership styles are then produced as follows:

1 *Authority-compliance management*, where the leader assumes a position of power by arranging work conditions efficiently and in so doing interferes minimally with the human elements.
2 *Team management*, where people are committed to accomplishing a task, group members are independent, and everyone holds a stake in an environment characterized by high trust, equality and respect.
3 *Country club management*, where the leader attempts to make all group members comfortable in a friendly atmosphere of work.
4 *Impoverished management*, where the leader extends limited effort in accomplishing the required work.
5 *Middle-of-the-road management*, where the leader attempts to balance behaviours that are task-oriented whilst retaining morale and drive amongst group members.

✐ Activity 19.2

1 Where would you place yourself on the Blake and Mouton leadership grid. Are you:

   (a) high/low in your concern for people?
   (b) high/low in your concern for production?

2 Which of the five styles applies to you?
3 For each of the five management styles, think of at least one individual, not necessarily in health care, who manages in this way.
4 Which of these management styles is the most appropriate in health care?

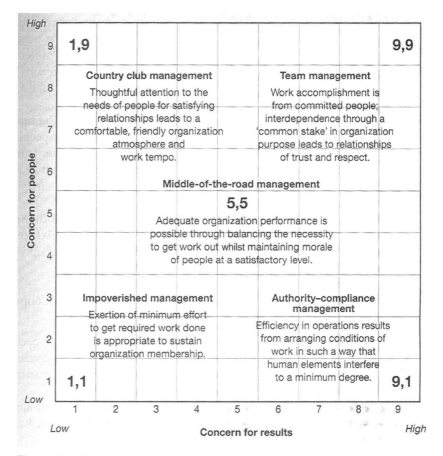

Figure 19.1 The Blake-Mouton leadership grid
Source: Blake and Mouton (1985)

Feedback

The 'team management' style is the one which encourages the active participation of health care professionals. However, there will be circumstances when 'authority-compliance' works better. Think of the people you identified as adopting the different styles, and think about which are the most effective. You will probably find it is the team management style. If your own style is not that of team management then you could consider using the team manager you identified as a role model.

Matching leadership styles to different situations

In the literature on managerial leadership, considerable time is usually devoted to what are termed *contingency theories*, in which the emphasis is on linking successful leaders to a particular situation, and identifying winning combinations. As you learnt in Chapter 4, contingency theories are based on the belief that there is no single style of leadership that is appropriate to all situations. For the remainder of this chapter, you will consider the use and application of three key contingency models in the health care context.

Fiedler's contingency theory

Fiedler (1967) argues that leadership behaviour is dependent upon the *favourability* of the leadership situation. In the model, Fiedler developed a 'least preferred co-worker' (LPC) scale (see Figure 19.2) asking leaders to rank the relationship between themselves and co-workers on a sliding eight-point scale indicating whether the relationship was very favourable (a high score) or very unfavourable (a low score).

Pleasant	· _·_·_·	· _·_·_·	Unpleasant
	8 7 6 5	4 3 2 1	
Friendly	· · · ·	· · · ·	Unfriendly
	8 7 6 5	4 3 2 1	
Quarrelsome	· · · ·	· · · ·	Harmonious
	1 2 3 4	5 6 7 8	
Cold	· · · ·	· · · ·	Warm
	1 2 3 4	5 6 7 8	
Accepting	· · · ·	· · · ·	Rejecting
	8 7 6 5	4 3 2 1	
Distant	· · · ·	· · · ·	Close
	1 2 3 4	5 6 7 8	
Helpful	· · · ·	· · · ·	Frustrating
	8 7 6 5	4 3 2 1	
Relaxed	· · · ·	· · · ·	Tense
	8 7 6 5	4 3 2 1	
Unenthusiastic	· · · ·	· · · ·	Enthusiastic
	1 2 3 4	5 6 7 8	
Rejecting	· · · ·	· · · ·	Accepting
	1 2 3 4	5 6 7 8	

Figure 19.2 An example of Fiedler's 'Least Preferred Co-Worker' (LPC) scales
Source: Fiedler (1967)

Figure 19.2 describes ten typical relationship-based items (but could include many more). By totalling the scores for each co-worker or group, Fiedler argued that a high score reflected a leader who enjoyed inter-personal communications and was motivated by acting in a supportive and considerate manner. Conversely, a low score signified a leader who derived more satisfaction from achieving tasks and who would be less motivated by the relational aspects to leadership. The score, therefore, reflected the manager's personal style of leadership.

Fiedler suggested that three variables determined the favourability of leadership in an organization:

1 *Leader–member relations* – the degree to which the leader is liked and trusted;
2 *The task structure* – the degree to which a role or action is clearly defined;
3 *Position power* – the degree to which a leader can exercise power by virtue of his or her position in the organization.

Fiedler constructed eight combinations of these group-task situations (Figure 19.3) that could be combined with scores for leadership style to determine whether leadership was either *very favourable* or *very unfavourable* or *moderately favourable* (mixed). Fiedler argued that a direct, controlling style of leadership worked better at the two extremes but that where a mixed picture emerged a more facilitative and participative mode of leadership was required to gain best results.

✏ Activity 19.3

Think of an individual or group who you lead in your health care organization or think of the leaders in your organization and their relationship with a certain group.

1 Using Fiedler's contingency model, would you say your health care organization's situation is:

(a) very favourable?
(b) very unfavourable?

2 If Fiedler is correct, should health care managers be:

(a) more relationship-oriented?
(b) more task-oriented?

Write down two reasons why this may be true.

↻ Feedback

1 In health care, at senior levels, 'leader–member relations' are often poor. There is a divide between clinicians and managers, with clinicians suspicious of the power they perceive managers to have and vice versa. In many situations the degree of task structure is low. And, as you saw previously, there is little positional power. The situation is therefore *very unfavourable*.

2 According to Fiedler, a task-oriented leader will perform better than a relationship-oriented one. You may have included the following reasons.

(a) Relationship-oriented leaders become de-motivated and de-energized when faced with unremitting hostility.
(b) In the short term, clinicians can often not be persuaded to act in the best interests of the organization if this conflicts with the best interests of their own or of their patients. If it is necessary to curtail their activity they may respond only to actions like the removal of resources (e.g. beds). This kind of action requires task-oriented leaders.

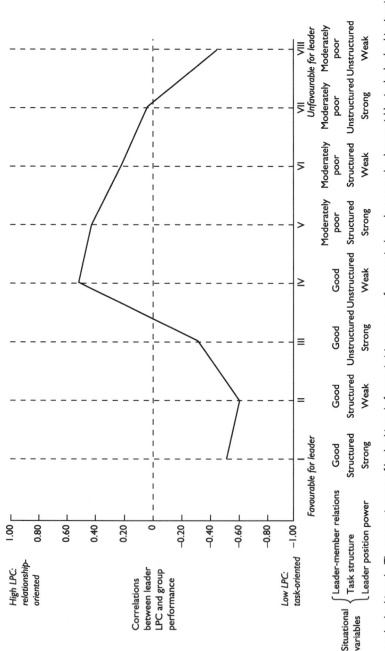

Figure 19.3 Correlations between leader's LPC scores and group effectiveness

Source: Fiedler (1967)

— = leadership style. The appropriateness of leadership style for maximizing group performance is dependent upon the three variables in the leadership situation.

(c) Task-oriented leaders do not spend time finding out what other people's goals are but concentrate on their own. Relationship-oriented leaders try to accommodate the aspirations of other people. In health care this may prove so complex that they become bogged down and lose sight of their own goals.

Path-goal theory

A second contingency model of leadership is the path-goal theory of House (1971). This model is based on the assumptions that an individual's motivation is based upon the expectation of delivering a successful outcome. Hence, performance is related to the extent to which a leader fulfils expectations. It has similar roots to *expectancy* theory which you examined in Chapter 14 in the context of performance-related pay.

House identified four main types of leadership:

1 *Directive leadership* manifests in telling subordinates what is expected of them and giving specific directions and tasks.
2 *Supportive leadership* involves a friendly and approachable concern to the need of others – or 'consideration' in the Ohio model described earlier.
3 *Participative leadership* involves consultation and evaluation of opinions before decisions are made.
4 *Achievement-oriented leadership* sets challenges, seeks improvement and shows confidence in the ability of others to do well.

Path-goal theory suggests that leaders should use one of the three styles depending on the personal characteristics of the subordinate (how they might react to the leader) and the nature of the task (whether it is simple or routine, or complex and unstructured).

Activity 19.4

Using Table 19.1, identify and reflect on a range of situations in which you as team leader used these styles or in which your team leader used these styles.

Table 19.1 Situations requiring different leadership styles

	Leadership style			
	Supportive	Directive	Achievement-oriented	Participative
Situation where this style worked well (preferably in your own experience)				
Impact on staff members concerned				
Outcome				

○↻ **Feedback**

The situations you have described will be unique to your experience. However, in path-goal relationships, when a task is highly structured and goals readily apparent, then leaders should not give directions or over-manage a situation. However, when a task is unstructured and the goals unclear, more directive leadership is welcomed. You may have found examples of both. According to the theory, effective leadership is based on both the willingness of the leader to help others in terms of direction and support, and the needs and willingness of others to want to be helped.

Hersey and Blanchard's situational leadership theory

Hersey and Blanchard's (1993) situational leadership theory grew out of the Ohio State model and can be visualized in Figure 19.4. A major component of the theory is that different managerial styles need to be adopted according to the task readiness of the people that the leader is attempting to influence. The level of readiness (or maturity) has four levels:

- *R1 – low follower readiness*, where followers lack commitment and motivation and may be unwilling and/or unable.
- *R2 – low/moderate follower readiness*, where followers can be motivated to make an effort but lack ability; in other words, willing but unable.
- *R3 – moderate/high follower readiness*, where followers are able and have the ability to perform but are unwilling or less ready to apply their ability.
- *R4 – high follower readiness*, where followers are both able and willing, committed to the task.

For each of the four levels, it is argued that the most appropriate style of leadership is related to a combination of 'task' and 'relationship' behaviour. Task behaviour is the extent to which the leader provides direction for the actions of followers, for example through setting goals and protocols for delivery. Relationship behaviour is the extent to which the leader engages in two-way communication with followers, for example to discuss options or examine stakeholders' views.

The combination of task and relationship behaviours derives four leadership styles:

- *S1 – telling*, where leaders provide guidance or orders to be performed but do not engage in close relationships with staff. This style of leadership is most appropriate where an employee has low follower readiness (R1).
- *S2 – selling*, where leaders 'sell' a direct task through engaging with staff, an approach most suited to moderate follower readiness (R2).
- *S3 – participating*, which emphasizes a high amount of two-way communication with no prescribed guidance, an approach most suited to moderate to high follower readiness (R3).
- *S4 – delegation*, where leaders provide little direction to staff since they are already motivated, competent and mature, an approach most suited to high follower readiness (R4).

According to Hersey and Blanchard (1993), the model draws attention to the different leadership styles that need to be adopted with different stakeholders or staff members reflecting their level of maturity, knowledge and willingness to work to organizational goals and tasks.

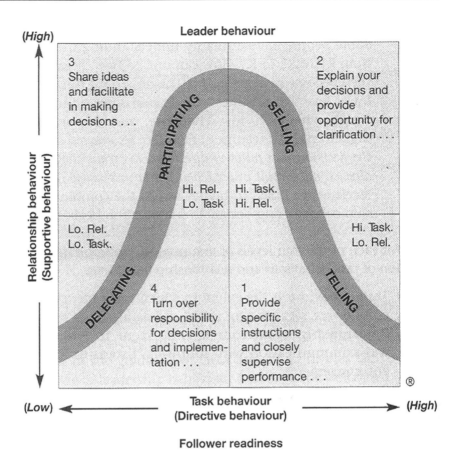

Figure 19.4 The situational leadership model

Source: Hersey (1984) cited in Mullins (1999)

✏️ **Activity 19.5**

1 Think of the members of your own team. Are they high or low in 'task readiness'?
2 According to Figure 19.4, which leadership style should you adopt for each of them?
3 Is your own task readiness high or low?

4   Which leadership style should your line managers adopt with you?
5   How could you encourage them to do so?

You may find it helpful to envisage a situation in which you will meet your team members (individually) over the next few days. Imagine adopting the leadership style you have identified as the most appropriate. How could you put into practice your suggestions in response to Question 4?

Feedback

It is likely that you, as a leader, will have a predominant style that may or may not be suitable for dealing with certain situations. It is worth finding out where your pre-dominant style lies, since this may help you identify your weaker leadership capabilities that need to be developed. Hence, if you predominantly use a direct 'telling' approach, this model suggests that its use with a senior clinician holding high positional power is unlikely to be the best approach. Moreover, if you prefer a 'facilitative' approach to management, the model suggests that the least senior members of a team often work better to structured directives since they need direction and may lack the maturity and knowledge to contribute to participative decision-making. Managers working in health care organizations, or across health and social care, often lack the power of direct command (or the knowledge of the best approach to take) and so must use participating styles of leadership to engage stakeholders in the design of service delivery methods.

Differences between models of contingency theory

According to Fiedler's theory, the style a leader adopts is fixed and he or she will always behave in that way. Hersey and Blanchard, however, suggest that leaders can choose their style according to the skills and confidence of their followers. Similarly the path-goal theory is based on the principle that these types of behaviours can be adopted by any leader, depending on the situation.

Summary

You have seen how trait, behavioural and contingency theories all help you to play to your strengths, to build in means of compensating for your weaknesses and, where you have a choice, to choose situations where you are most likely to succeed. However, often you will not be able to choose the team or the situation you are asked to manage. In these cases, it is important to remember that you can select your behaviour or leadership style; and the Hersey–Blanchard and path-goal theories provide a means of diagnosing which style will be most effective.

References

Blake, R. and Mouton, J. (1985) *The New Managerial Grid III: The Key to Leadership Excellence*. Houston: Gulf Publishing Co.

Fiedler, F. (1967) *A Theory of Leadership Effectiveness*. New York: McGraw-Hill.

Fleishman, E. (1974) Leadership climate, human relations training and supervisory behaviour, in E. Fleishman and A. Bass. (eds) *Studies in Personnel and Industry Psychology*, 3rd edn. New York: Dorsey.

Hersey, P. and Blanchard, K. (1993) *Management of Organizational Behaviour: Utilizing Human Resources*, 6th edn. London: Prentice-Hall.

House, R. (1971) A path-goal theory of leadership effectiveness, *Administrative Science Quarterly*, 16: 321–38.

Mullins, L.J. (1999) *Management and Organizational Behaviour*. London: Financial Times Pitman Publishing, 5th edn.

Glossary

7S model This model suggests that there are seven aspects of an organization that need to be in harmony with each other: strategy, structure, systems, staff, style, shared values and skills.

Analogy Making decisions about staffing by considering the structure of another health care organization.

Appraisal Assessment of the performance of personnel within an organization based on specified standards and procedures.

Appraisal interview A meeting between a member of staff (appraisee) and his or her appraiser, to discuss the appraisee's performance, expectations and prospects within the organization.

Assessment centre approach An approach to filling a staff post that combines several selection methods.

Autocratic leadership Leaders make decisions on behalf of their staff.

Behavioural approaches Theories that suggest it is not personality but particular behaviours that determine whether or not a leader is successful.

Benchmarking The process of comparing performance against that of the leaders in a particular industry or against targets.

Business process re-engineering The fundamental rethinking and radical redesign of business processes to achieve dramatic improvements in performance such as cost, quality, service and speed.

Capacity A measure of the maximum possible output that an organizational unit can achieve over a given time period.

Capacity utilization A measure of the extent to which the potential maximum capacity of an organization is being used.

Capitation payments A prospective means of paying health care staff based on the number of people they provide care for.

Career development The development of staff members' careers within an organization. The acquisition of skills and experience, enabling employees to attain more senior positions within the organization.

Career paths The normal routes of progression within an organization. They provide a source of information for employees to make choices about personal advancement, and for the organization they provide a way of ensuring that jobs relate to strategic goals, by identifying the key attributes post-holders should possess and how those attributes should be developed.

Classical management theory A scientifically based approach to the practice of management involving tasks and functions.

Coercive power Power to punish or to withhold rewards.

Community financing Collective action of local communities to finance health services through pooling out-of-pocket payments and ensuring services are accountable to the community.

Complicated easy management concepts Concepts that are mastered using intelligence and, once mastered, require only intelligence to implement.

Conceptual skill The ability of managers to understand the complexities and issues within an organization and the role and strength of management within it.

Contingency approaches Theories which suggest that different behaviours are required in different situations and that successful leaders are those who can move flexibly from one style to another as the situation changes.

Continuous change Change that is ongoing, evolving and cumulative.

Convergence/divergence Processes promoting similarities/differences between countries, or between private and public sector organizations.

Crowding-in A situation in which motivations of individuals to perform activities are increased by financial rewards.

Crowding-out A situation in which the professional or altruistic behaviours of individuals are adversely affected by direct remuneration for the task.

Decisional roles Managerial roles at the 'front line', including dealing with disputes, negotiating with staff, allocating resources and initiating change.

Democratic (participative) leadership Leadership whereby staff are involved in making decisions.

Developmental change Change that enhances or corrects existing aspects of an organization.

Diagnosis related group (DRG) Classification system that assigns patients to categories on the basis of the likely cost of their episode of hospital care. Used as basis for determining level of prospective payment by purchaser.

Discrimination The tendency to give preference to one gender (usually men) or to one ethnic group, disregarding the merits of other groups (e.g. women).

Emergent change Change that is apparently spontaneous and/or unplanned.

Employment relations Management of the relationship between the organization and its staff as a whole.

Empowerment The development of decision-making abilities amongst people at all levels in the organization.

Episodic change Change that happens infrequently as an organization or system moves from one strategy to the next.

Essential package of care A strategy for purchasing services that achieve the greatest reduction in the burden of disease with available resources.

Expectancy theory A theory suggesting that the level of performance is directly related to the level of individual reward.

Expert power Power resulting from specialist skills or knowledge.

Favouritism The tendency to ignore considerations of merit by giving preference to members of one's own family, ethnic group or geographical region, or to individuals favoured for some other personal reason.

Fee-for-service A means of paying health care staff on the basis of the actual items of care provided.

Force field analysis Can be used to identify individual and environmental 'forces' that may help or hinder the successful implementation of change.

Group think The way members of a group distort their thinking to become overly supportive of suggestions made within the group and dismissive of suggestions and challenges that come from outside it.

Human resource development Activities that aim to improve the capacity and quality of the workforce, employee relations, equal opportunities and staff motivation.

Human resource strategy The overall plan for the treatment of staff in an organization.

Human skill The ability of managers to work with and through people, including the abilities to lead and to motivate.

Informational roles Managerial roles based on fulfilling interpersonal goals, including monitoring activity, disseminating information and dealing with the concerns of key stakeholders.

Instrumental work motivation A situation in which workers value work principally for the material rewards it provides.

Interpersonal roles Managerial roles based on formal authority, including leadership, liaison with external organizations and acting as a figurehead.

Intrinsic work motivation A situation in which work is valued for itself rather than for its material rewards.

Job analysis The process of determining the content of jobs and the kinds of skills needed for performing them.

Job description A description of the job, including its main purpose, responsibilities and key tasks.

Leadership A relationship through which one person influences the behaviour and actions of other people.

Legitimate power Power given by an organization, or by a statutory framework, to tell subordinates what to do. Subordinates accept this as legitimate.

Loans (grants, donations) External aid used to fund care services, usually with a set of conditions attached.

Managerial competencies Specifically developed criteria based on the key managerial skills (technical, human and conceptual) required for a particular job.

Managerial judgement Decision-making on the basis of specific criteria developed for the purpose when precedent and analogy are not helpful; ideally a needs-based approach that takes into account historically developed structures and stakeholders' interests.

Mission statement A statement expressing the purpose of an organization, department or individual. It should convey a clear sense of direction and form the basis for day-to-day decisions.

Nepotism The granting of special consideration to members of one's own family.

New public management An approach to government involving the application of private sector management techniques.

Organizational learning A transformational process that seeks to help organizations develop and use knowledge to change and improve themselves on an ongoing basis.

Out-of-pocket (direct) payments Payment made by a patient to a provider.

Performance The process of achieving aims both at the organizational level and with respect to contributions to those aims at the level of work units and individual staff.

Performance indicators Financial and non-financial measures used for monitoring activity levels, efficiency and quality of service provision by comparing actual with expected results.

Performance management A systematic approach to the management of individual performance, seeing it in the context of the overall strategy of the organization.

Performance-related pay A system that provides financial incentives to individuals and/or groups to work more effectively to meet measurable goals.

Person specification An outline of the abilities, qualifications and experience required of the job-holder, usually distinguishing between essential and desirable requirements.

Personal power Power arising from personality and behaviour. This power includes expert and referent power.

Person-oriented organizational culture A professional culture in which the organization has no intrinsic value beyond the growth, development and self-realization of its members.

PESTELI A checklist for making sure all relevant aspects of the environment in which the organization is operating are considered.

Planned change Change that is a product of conscious reasoning and action.

Position power Power people have because of the position they hold in an organization. It includes legitimate, reward and coercive power.

Positive action The inclusion of a positive statement of non-discrimination in advertising for applicants, or providing special arrangements such as flexi-time, nurseries or job-sharing for workers with young children.

Positive discrimination Selection that favours people from a disadvantaged group.

Power-oriented organizational culture Attitudes tending towards aggression and exploitation within organizations that are autocratic and controlled from the top.

Precedent An approach to decision-making about staffing needs based on previous custom and practice.

Private health insurance Voluntary insurance to cover health care costs based on the individual's level of risk.

Problem-solving method A framework upon which all management practices are built, consisting of problem identification, problem definition, problem analysis, developing solutions and recommending actions.

Process modelling A way of understanding how a current situation works and providing a clear articulation of how a new one is to be different by capturing visually the dynamics of the situation so that they can be discussed with all those involved.

Productivity A measure of how efficiently inputs are converted into outputs.

Prospective payment Paying providers before any care is delivered, based on predefined activity levels and anticipated costs.

Purchasing The process by which funds are used to pay providers.

Quality Those features or characteristics of a product or service that demonstrate 'fitness for purpose' relating to their ability to meet stated needs.

Quality chain The chain of suppliers and customers of health services. The integrity of the chain is important for ensuring service quality is upheld.

Recruitment and selection The process of finding suitable staff to carry out the jobs identified as necessary for an organization.

Referent power Power that comes from personality characteristics which command identification, respect or admiration.

Retrospective payment Paying providers for any work they have undertaken, with no agreement in advance.

Revenue collection The process by which a health system receives money.

Reward power Power resulting from the ability to give rewards.

Risk pooling A way in which revenue is managed to ensure that the risk of having to pay for health care is borne by all rather than by the individual.

Role theory A role-based analysis of managerial tasks, originating with the work of Mintzberg, which examines observed roles as opposed to prescribed tasks.

Role-oriented organizational culture A setting in which the correct response tends to be more highly valued than the effective one, within typically bureaucratic organizations that are slow to adapt to change.

Simple hard management concepts Concepts that are simple to understand but require courage and discipline to implement.

Social health insurance Compulsory contributions to a health insurance fund gaining individual or group entitlement to health care benefits – usually based on employer and employee contributions.

Soft systems methodology Articulation of complex social processes in a participatory way, allowing people's viewpoints to be brought to light, challenged and tested.

Stability rate A measure of how well a staff category is standing up to erosion in its numbers due to wastage from the organization.

Staff turnover Staff wastage, or changes in staff levels over time; they can be due either to avoidable circumstances (such as dissatisfaction with poor management) or to unavoidable events (such as retirement, illness).

Stakeholders Those involved in a selection process who can affect, or are affected by, the appointment.

Strategic fit This occurs when the organization's goals (mission) are achievable given its resources and its environment.

Strategic management The process of analysis and decision-making that is concerned with ensuring strategic fit.

Strategic purchasing The identification and procurement of the best care to meet the goals for the health care system.

Superordinate goals The highest goals of an organization; fundamental desired outputs that enable managers to assess performance relative to its mission.

SWOT analysis The SWOT (strengths-weaknesses-opportunities-threats) analysis is a framework for analysing the fit between the mission, the resources and the environment. The purpose of a SWOT is to identify the critical issues an organization must address if it is to achieve its mission.

Task-oriented organizational culture Achievement and effectiveness are valued above the demands of authority or procedure within organizations whose structure is adaptive to tasks or functions, and emphasis is placed on rapid and flexible response to change conditions.

Taxation A method of financing health care and other public services based on either a direct payroll or income taxes, or indirect tax on goods and services.

Technical skill The ability of a manager to use knowledge, methods, techniques and equipment necessary for the performance of a specific task.

Total quality management (continuous quality improvement) An approach to quality improvement that involves the commitment of all members of an organization to meeting the needs of its external and internal customers.

Training specification An account of the knowledge and skills (technical and social) the post-holder needs to perform the job satisfactorily.

Trait theories Theories which suggest that leaders with certain personality traits will be more successful than others.

Transformational change Change that is accepted by an organization as a norm so that a continuous improvement cycle of adaptation is developed.

Tribalism The tendency of members in a profession to engage in a phenomenon known as group think.

Whole systems thinking An approach in which issues, forces and actions are not seen as isolated phenomena but part of a connected system of activity.

Index

Page numbers in *italics* refer to figures and tables.

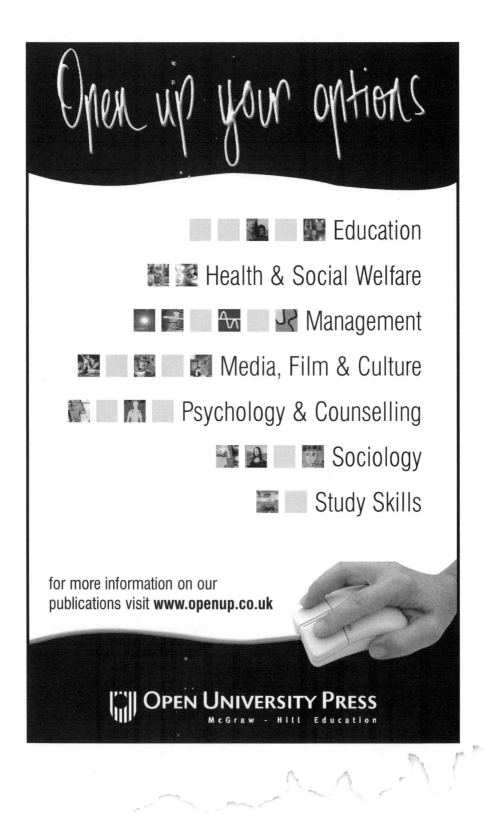